Wow! What a Ride!
A Journey with Cancer

WOW! WHAT A RIDE!
A JOURNEY WITH CANCER

BY CELLA BOSMA

DORDT COLLEGE PRESS

Layout and cover design by Carla Goslinga

Copyright © 2010 by Jerry Bosma

Printed in the United States of America.

Dordt College Press   www.dordt.edu/dordt_press
498 Fourth Avenue NE
Sioux Center, Iowa 51250
United States of America

ISBN: 978-0-932914-84-2

The Library of Congress Cataloging-in-Publication Data is on file with the Library of Congress, Washington, D.C.

Library of Congress Control Number: 2010921372

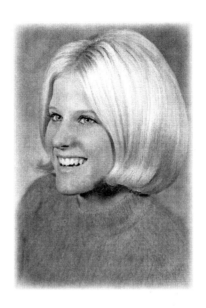

DEDICATION

*We dedicate this CaringBridge Journal to the
hundreds of students, colleagues, friends, and relatives
from all over the world who, with their words, cards,
visits, guest book entries, and above all, prayers,
walked with Cella on her journey with cancer.*

Cella's family

PREFACE

"No man is an island, entire of itself; every man is a piece of the continent. . . .

Any man's death diminishes me, because I am involved in Mankind; and therefore never send to know for whom the bell tolls; it tolls for thee" (Meditation 17, John Donne). Donne's comment suggests not merely that a death should remind everyone of his or her own mortality, but also that each of us should ask "Why not me ?"

More than anything else, this book is a meditation on a Christian's dying of cancer in the 21st century. But it also gives us a specific instance of how the death of one human being can "diminish" the lives of others. The tolling of church bells once alerted us to this fact. Some may have lived in areas where church bells rang at all funerals, once for a one-year-old's death, 50 times for a 50-year-old's death. I have heard such bells; most people hearing it could not help but feel "diminished."

For Cella Bosma the bell tolled first when she heard her doctor say, "You have cancer." But Cella believed she had a fighting chance to delay or even to ward off the sentence. She believed in the power of prayer, she had hundreds praying for her, and she had modern medicine as an ally.

Both Cella and later the family wondered, "Why Cella?"/"Why not me?" As Os Guinness in his book *Unspeakable* writes, "At the deepest level, the question of 'Why me?' probes the frightening thought of ultimate chaos and the terror of randomness." But both Cella and the family believe a loving God is in control, though the questions why or why not remain a mystery amid the cries and prayers of God's people. As believers they would say, as Guinness suggests, "Father, I do not understand you but I trust you" (p.71).

This story shows us Cella whose abundance of both faith and courage were strong allies of her tenacious love of life. Some, when told they have cancer, choose to slink away, to "hole up," feeling unjustly gypped and wanting above all to be left alone. Cella, on the other hand, took her "sentence" to the Christian community for which she had for decades been an agent of love and comfort.

For more than two years she wrote of her fears, needs, hopes, and occasional frustrations while receiving X-rays, MRIs, PET scans, EKGs, chemotherapy, radiation, meds for cancer and then meds to control side effects of other meds. Meanwhile, she received visits, cards, and e-mails of support and comfort by the hundreds, most of them assuring her of the fervent prayers of friends and relatives from across at least three continents.

Yet, as she and her family said, they felt as if she was on a roller coaster—good news one day, scary news the next—while always hearing in the wind the tolling of death's bell, at times softly, at times more persistently.

Cella's CaringBridge entries during the two years of her battle show some swings in mood, but reveal hope, faith, and love to the end. Reading it, you will hear the knell of death against the persistent drumbeat of faith.

To conclude, to those of us who wonder with Cella and her family, "Why Cella?" we can recall the deaths of others of whom we may have asked, "Why does God take any Kingdom servant who meets God's apparent needs on earth so effectively? Why did He not protect the first disciples who had their lives cut short for sharing the gospel?" In the end we leave such mysteries to our Creator God.   mvb

THE BEGINNING

Cella's journey began on Wednesday, January 17, 2007 when she had a breast lump checked at her family practice doctor. She had a biopsy the same day, the results the following day, a mastectomy Monday, January 22 at 8 a.m. Everything happened very fast. We were still processing Cella's twin sister Marcia Rozeboom's breast cancer, which was diagnosed shortly before Christmas. We are still processing all of the emotions and information from the last week.

Surgery went well. The surgeon found cancer in the breast and in the lymph system. The night of the surgery, Cella passed out on her way to the bathroom, falling on her incision site. On Wednesday, January 24, Cella had another surgery to remove over a quart of excess blood that had clotted at the incision site. Because of the loss of blood, Cella's hemoglobin dropped to eight and left her feeling very tired.

Cella was discharged on Thursday, January 25. Before discharge, the surgeon reported that he removed twenty-seven lymph nodes, seven of those being cancerous. Even with the high number of lumps, the doctor was hopeful that cancer may not have travelled to other parts of her body. Monday, January 29, Cella returned to have her drain site removed. We hope soon to have results from the scans they have done (and will do) to determine if the cancer has travelled to her lungs, liver, or bone marrow.

We were reminded by the words of Roy Lessin to "be assured that regardless of where we are, what you are doing or what you are going through, in all ways God is doing the most loving thing concerning us." It is with that assurance that we confidently begin to walk this journey of breast cancer.

They are not sure if the nodules are cancerous or not, so they are possibly going to do a PET scan of her whole body to get more details. All of this will depend on what Dr. Krie, the oncologist, says on Friday. Cella will also talk to Dr. Krie about whether to have another mastectomy and explore her options further. She will be having a bone scan tomorrow at 11:00 a.m. and will be meeting with her oncologist on Friday morning.

January/February 2007

Tuesday, January 30, 2007 7:59 a.m.

This morning I woke up and found many emotions running through me as I read the encouraging remarks in the guest book. I was humbled, encouraged, rejuvenated, joyful, and more. I was also reminded of who God is through the faithfulness of His people. I was astounded at the breadth of God's kingdom and the depth of God's love. I want to thank my two lovely daughters, Megan and Mindy, for all their work in putting the site together. What a blessing they have been and continue to be! (Josh blesses me in other ways.)

Jerry continues to be wonderfully supportive and even though all of this has made him extremely busy, he keeps on encouraging and helping me.

As Mindy wrote last night, I will be having the bone scan done today. If you find a few minutes to pray, please pray that I can stand the long lie on the skinny board.

I've already written this to a few of you, but I wanted quickly to share the challenge the words of Philippians 1:21 have brought to me. Paul is writing from prison and he says, "For to me, to live is Christ and to die is gain." I'm looking forward to the gain I will receive one day as a child of God, but I am thankful that the prognosis right now doesn't say death. So that means I live and with that living I, like Paul, must live in Christ. That is my challenge—to live through this trial always living as Christ would, something I can't do completely, but I hope with God's grace, can do in part. This is my prayer.

Wednesday, January 31, 2007 9:21 a.m.

"Satisfy us in the morning with your unfailing love, that we may sing for joy and be glad all our days" (Psalm 90:14).

"I trust in you, O Lord; I say, 'You are my God. My times are in your hands" (Psalm 31:14-15).

Jesus said, " . . . do not worry about tomorrow, for tomorrow will worry about itself. Each day has enough trouble of its own'" (Matthew 6:34).

These are the verses I came across this morning to make me think—

"This is the day the Lord has made; let us rejoice and be glad in it."

Today I am rejoicing in the blessing of great friends and family. I'm enjoying the beautiful flowers that many of you sent. And I'm thanking God for all the advancements that have been made in the medical field. Yesterday I had a bone scan. What an amazing machine. It was a long process but one that should be able to give information about cancer cells but also information concerning my hip that has been giving me problems for some time. I'm tired today, but as I see the snow fly, I'm glad I can stay indoors and rest. My next appointment will be on Friday when I see the oncologist. Thanks for all your prayers and warm wishes. You help give me strength to face each day. Thanks.

Thursday, February 1, 2007 9:42 a.m.

The thought of going to the oncologist tomorrow has been weighing heavy on my mind, but this morning I was led to read a passage on waiting for results. The author reminded me that God already holds the test results in his hands, and that because we belong to Him, everything will somehow work together for good. Two verses were helpful to me: "I will praise the Lord, who counsels me; even at night my heart instructs me. I have set the Lord always before me. Because he is at my right hand, I will not be shaken" (Psalm 16:7-8). "Who of you by worrying can add a single hour to his life? Since you cannot do this very little thing, why do you worry about the rest?" (Luke 12:25-26). And then I read Greg Anderson's "Always choose hope." I am holding onto the hope of a good report tomorrow and yet I know that whatever comes, I have a mighty God who will carry us through. Thanks to all of you who have written (and signed in). Your words and promise of prayers encouraged me greatly.

Friday, February 2, 2007 6:54 a.m.

Last night was a sleepless night. I finally got up and did some work and then decided to check the messages on this site. As always I was encouraged and strengthened by all my friends and family. It is wonderful to know that I am not traveling this road by myself—sorry to drag all of you into this. Psalm 4:8 did quiet my spirit and help me focus. I need to rest in the realization that whatever happens, I can rely on God to carry us through. Your words of encouragement help tremendously. I am humbled by your words of kindness along with your willingness to pray and help me bear this burden. Thank you and please help me pray that what we hear today will be bearable and lead to recovery.

Friday, February 2, 2007 1:59 p.m.

Well, I'm back from the oncologist. But before I say more, I have to tell you how much you have all helped bear the news. Your reminders to me that you are lifting me up in prayer and that my strength comes from and is in God will help as we face the next week. The oncologist was very honest with us and didn't hold back any possible diagnosis. She laid out our worst fears and told us of lesser possibilities. I must say I wasn't quite prepared to hear what could be ahead. The important thing now is for me (actually all of us) not to jump ahead to conclusions.

My morning began by developing a leak. (I sound like a balloon!) One of my stitches loosened and I found myself bleeding all over the bathroom. After a frantic call to Jerry, I called the doctor and he assured me that my incision was draining and that I'd be okay. Good words to hear. Dr. Krie, the oncologist, was very honest with us and told us of her concerns. The major concern right now is the lung. She feels that the spots are a concern so she set up a PET scan for me on Tuesday, along with a biopsy of the lung. I'll have the results of the PET scan already on Tuesday and the biopsy by Friday.

She talked about treatment plans, but the result of the lung tests will determine which route she will take. To be honest with you, this isn't what I was hoping to hear. The words that cancer may be outside the breast area scared me. I don't really feel like going through this. I want to be back in school doing what I love to do. But for now, this is reality. I know in my heart that God will carry us through but right now, not knowing is really difficult. Please pray with us that we can have a calm spirit while we wait for further results. Thanks much for your support and your prayers. I don't know where I'd be without all of you. I trust you will continue to lift us up in prayer.

Saturday, February 3, 2007 7:57 a.m.

How wonderful a good night's sleep feels—another assurance that the prayers of God's people are being answered.

When I woke up this morning, the song "This is the Day" was singing in my head. First of all it reminded me of singing this song at a wedding that my sister and I sang at (yes, we were the soloists!) over Christmas break. We did not produce the most beautiful sound, but the bride and groom didn't seem to care. They smiled throughout the whole song, and so did we. This was their special day, and they enjoyed every minute of it. Today is a day given to us by God. It may not seem as special as a wedding day, but to God it is just as important that we honor Him today.

As I feel somewhat freeze-framed until I learn more about my diagnosis, I look to Psalm 90:12: "Teach us to number our days aright, that we may gain a heart of wisdom." What a way to remember to love each day because, no matter what it brings, God gives us this day and He will be with us in it. I feel God walking beside me—especially through all of your calls, cards, CaringBridge messages, and e-mails. Thank you. I hope that each of you feels His presence in you today too.

Sunday, February 4, 2007 8:25 a.m.

Good Morning,

As I saw the sunrise this morning, I was reminded of Lamentations 3:22: "Because of the Lord's great love we are not consumed, for his compassions never fail. They are new every morning; great is your faithfulness." I say to myself, "The Lord is my portion; therefore I will wait for him."

As sure as we are that each day the sun will rise, so sure are we that God will be faithful in His walk with us today. Trusting in God's faithfulness day by day makes us confident in His great promises for the future. I'm looking forward to attending church this morning and learning more about who God is and how I can put my trust in Him. Again, thanks very much for your encouragement and prayers. As Tuesday gets closer, we feel all the more need for prayers for patience, peace, and hope. I pray that all of you have a blessed day, communing with God, family, and friends.

Monday, February 5, 2007 8:47 a.m.

Good Morning,

Many of you who drop in on this site are probably already at work. It's been a lazy morning for me. I miss my work, my students, and my colleagues, but I am glad for the release from work that has been granted to me so graciously by the college. My colleagues have unselfishly picked up my workload for which I am thankful but at times struggle with what I have added to their already heavy load. They seem to have a much better handle on my ability to come back to work than I do. I'm grateful they were given wisdom and made plans for my classes. Even though I miss teaching tremendously, I know that my students are in very good hands and are getting the education that they have learned to expect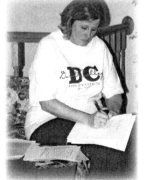

from the education department at Dordt. So, very humbly, I thank everyone who has helped pick up the extra work.

I must tell you that each time I read the entries in the guest book I weep, not with tears of sadness but tears of gratitude. Each entry encourages me and gives me strength and hope. Yesterday someone mentioned Psalm 23 as a Psalm that gave them courage, and it reminded me of one of the segments from Ray Vander Laan's series. He reminded us that the green pastures of the Psalm were not like the lush alfalfa fields we have in Iowa, but small green tufts that were sparse in the lands of Israel. When the shepherds of Israel led their sheep to the green, it probably wasn't a whole field, but a tuft of grass tucked between stones on sandy soil. The shepherd knew how to find that tuft that would bring nourishment and life. So it is with God. Sometimes the pasture doesn't look full of grass, but God is able to bring us to the place where we can find peace, rest, and nourishment.

I have found that your notes to me are like those tufts in the hardness of life. The words you have spoken to me and the passages you have quoted are my strength for my day. "The Lord is my shepherd, I shall not be in want."

Tuesday, February 6, 2007 6:48 a.m.

After a night of tossing and turning, we are ready to leave for the hospital. We stayed at Jerry's sister in Sioux Falls last night to save some travel this morning. We are leaving in a few minutes for the 7:30 PET scan; at noon we will go to Avera for the lung biopsy. As soon as I can, I'll try to update this site. We're praying for good results and for grace to accept the news we will hear today. Some of the results won't be back until Thursday or Friday. Thanks for your prayers—they are holding us strong.

Tuesday, February 6, 2007 12:35 p.m.

I talked to mom and we got great news. The PET scan went very well, and Dr. Krie said that she is going to treat mom for aggressive cancer and doesn't think that the lung is going to be a problem as of right now. How wonderful God is; we see the power of prayer. Thank you for all of your prayers. Mindy

Wednesday, February 7, 2007 8:20 a.m.

I'll try again. I wrote a lengthy journal last night and lost it as I submitted it. I was too tired to try again. Yesterday began at 7:00 a.m. by leaving Jerry's sister's house, where we had spent the night, for the PET scan clinic. It was snowy so we were glad that we had to drive only across town. At the clinic I was injected with a radioactive material and then required to lie as quietly as I could while the fluid did its job. (I knew there was a reason that I didn't sleep well the night before.) I wasn't allowed to do anything, not even read. I was told that the muscles I would use to hold the book could cause an inaccuracy in the test results. I was thankful for all the songs and scripture that I had been reminded of the past week in the guest book entries—I used this quiet time to relax and reflect on them.

After the wait, I spent about 45 minutes passing in and out of a tube. I have been very thankful for exceptionally kind and caring technicians who seem to care about one's comfort both physically and emotionally. From here we went to see Dr. Krie, the oncologist. We went into her office holding the pictures that would reveal what our life would/could look like for the next half year. We were prepared to hear anything.

I would have to say we were scared, but not terrified. We were confident that God's grace would flood us with what we needed just as we have experienced in the past. Dr. Krie had been very frank with us during our first visit so we knew that she would again tell us things as she saw them. Well, as you already know from Mindy's entry, we were blessed with the best news possible. Later we asked ourselves, do you think a week ago we would rejoice with the diagnosis of breast cancer? How much better those words sounded than breast cancer on the lung. This she called curable!

All I could think of was Praise God and Thank You Lord! The song that the Cary Christian staff almost always sings for us when we are in Mississippi rang through my head. ("Praise God . . ." to the tune of "Amazing Grace.") Thanks for the memory, CC staff. Neither Jerry nor I could stop smiling. We were very thankful for the good news. The doctor remains cautious, but very hopeful that the cancer stayed contained in the breast and lymph nodes. From her office, we went to Avera Hospital for the lung biopsy. They still wanted to get a better picture of what is on my lung. They were a little unsure about being able to get the needle into the right spot on the lung, but Dr. Small did a great job of finding the spot and extracting threads of material from it. After this I was required to lie for 3-4 hours and then take a lung x-ray to make sure the lung hadn't pulled away from the wall. What a blessing to find my cousin's wife on duty and assigned to helping me. (I know Pat, just one more of my relatives.)

I was instructed to stay quiet for the evening and to stay in Sioux Falls in case there would be bleeding. The night went well and I feel great this morning. My sister, who works in Sioux Falls, will take me back to Iowa this afternoon. Wow. What a day! Thanks for sharing it with us by upholding us in prayer. We felt well-cared-for and felt God's presence throughout the day. He does work in wonderful ways.

So what does this mean for the future? I will begin chemo treatments as soon as I'm healed from the mastectomy. (By the way, the PET scan showed absolutely no cancerous tissue in my left breast.) We'll find out for sure on Monday, but it looks like I'll take eight treatments, two weeks apart. Then I'll go through a series of radiation. I'm not especially looking forward to this time, but I have been encouraged by many who have traveled this route and have assured me that this time passes quickly. The doctor is quite sure that I will be able to teach during this time, for which I am very grateful.

Psalm 100 comes to mind this morning. It was a Psalm that I taught to both second and fifth graders when I was teaching in elementary school. I loved that Psalm then, but now I hold it even dearer to my heart. "Shout for joy to the Lord—serve the Lord with gladness!" I am shouting Thank You, Lord. I pray that I can serve Him with gladness throughout these next trying months and in the future. Yes, the future! I look forward to each and every day.

Thursday, February 8, 2007 9:36 a.m.

Hi Ho Hi Ho, it's off to work—well, maybe not. It is more like Hi Ho Hi Ho, it's off to a medical facility. I thought I was done with testing but today I am scheduled for a test called MUGA. It is a scan of my heart to see if it can take the chemo treatments. Dr. Krie wants the test results by Monday so she can affirm what she will be proposing for treatment. Over the past 24 hours I've had a bit of pain as a result of the lung biopsy. I wasn't quite prepared for that but should have anticipated it I guess. When someone pulls a little out of one of your organs, I suppose pain is expected. Pain pills and not moving much is helping control the pain. I'm hoping to have Dr. Stelzer drain the surgical site once more today. I can tell that the collection of fluid is slowing down. That makes my incision area much more comfortable.

As I was reflecting on all that has happened in the whirlwind of the last few weeks, I was brought back to a sermon I heard John W. Cooper, a professor of philosophical theology at Calvin Seminary, preach about a year ago. He was looking at the brokenness of this world, the break in shalom, that all of us deal with and which for me at this time is the diagnosis of cancer. I don't want to bore you or take up too much of your time, but he said some powerful things that have helped me deal with those horrible things that happen in life. He said, in a nutshell, that we often feel a need to understand and make sense of evil. We want to know what benefit we will see from the pain we endure in our lives. John Cooper says we may not always see the "good" things that come from the "bad" things, but we will always see that God is with us, loving and sustaining us even through the greatest pain and darkest despair. He spoke about how "all things work for good" may not mean "each and every thing," but "most likely it means the totality of things." This means His whole plan works for the good of those who are called according to His purpose (Romans 8:28). This helps me to understand that I may still have to endure some tough times in life, but through it all, God is always with me, loving and keeping me, even through the sharpest pains in my life. Nothing ". . . will be able to separate us from the love of God that is in Christ Jesus our Lord" (Romans 8:39). John Cooper said, "God himself strengthens our faith, hope, and love, just as He did for Job." That is my comfort and I hope it is yours too.

Friday, February 9, 2007 10:03 a.m.

No doctors, no tests, no pokes today. Yesterday I had an EKG and a heart scan. These were done as precautionary measures to make sure that my heart is strong enough for the chemo treatments which will be described to us on Monday by Dr. Krie. By the way, for those of you who do not know Dr. Krie, she is a young woman doctor who recently moved to Sioux Falls from Iowa City. She satellites to Sioux Center. She is very up-to-date on breast cancer, honest, thorough, and caring. I am very thankful for her and for the other doctors who are helping me.

I had a great day yesterday. After my tests, I saw Dr. Stelzer who drained my surgical site again, and then I went to the office and talked with some of my colleagues. It felt good to be on campus, look at my clean office, talk with friends, and grab some books to study. It felt good to be independent, drive my VW Bug, and do my own thing. Jerry warned me that being "up and about" (that's how he puts it) could make me tired, but I was having so much fun I didn't notice until I got home. Wow! I was exhausted which allowed for a great night of sleep.

There is a devotional that I often read to my Methods of Bible class that has come to mean a lot to me. It is based on James 1:4: "Perseverance must finish its work so that you may be mature and complete, not lacking anything."

The devotional is a fantasy story about a couple who come across a tea cup in a fancy store in England. As they are commenting on the cup, it begins to speak. It tells of its journey in becoming a beautiful work of art. The cup began as a lump of clay and after lots of hard rolling, it was placed on a spinning wheel, then put in a hot oven. The maker painted the cup with a horrible smelling paint which made the tea cup sick. Once again the cup was put in a hot oven, one that was even hotter this time. All the while the tea cup begged for the maker to stop, but the maker continually said, "Not yet." Just when the cup thought it could take no more, the process was completed and the cup was allowed to look at itself in a mirror. The cup responded with, "Why, that can not be me. What I am seeing is something beautiful." The maker replied, "I know it hurt to be rolled and patted, but if I had left you, you would have dried up. I know it made you dizzy to spin around on the wheel, but if I had stopped, you would have crumbled. I know it hurt, and it was hot and disagreeable in the oven, but if I hadn't put you there, you would have cracked. I know the fumes were bad when I brushed and painted you all over, but if I hadn't done that, you never would have hardened. You wouldn't have had any color in your life, and if I hadn't put you back in the second oven, you wouldn't have survived for very long because the hardness wouldn't have held. Now you are what I had in mind when I first began with you." As each of us faces trials in our lives, we can be comforted to know that God is working in us. As we yell out, "Let me out," He often says, "Not yet," and continues to groom us for the person He longs for us to be: "he who began a good work in you will carry it on to completion until the day of Christ Jesus" (Philippians 1:6).

Friday, February 9, 2007 10:04 a.m.

I forgot to add this before I submitted my journal entry this morning. I'll probably not journal again until I hear my results on Monday. I do want to thank all of you again for the many ways you have encouraged me. God has surely used you in wonderful ways to lift up my family and me. We've loved the flowers, the books, the food, the lotions, the figurines, the cards and messages. All of them have shown us the power of the communion of God's people. It is humbling! Have a wonderful weekend!

Sunday, February 11, 2007 5:34 p.m.

Hello my dear friends,

I thought I would probably not update my journal until Monday but I've been so overwhelmed by the generosity of many of you that I had to write today to say once again, "Thank you." I continue to be astonished and surprised by the many greetings and acts of kindness that have been shown to us. Some of you have written very encouraging notes; I'm often surprised when I see the signature on cards and I think—I can't believe they too remembered me. Some of you I know well, and I thank you for your encouragement, but some of you I've never met and I thank you too. All of this encouragement reminds me that we are not only in God's good hands, but in the wonderful hands of His people. I get such a warm feeling knowing that my family is also being supported by such good people.

I have a little true confession to make. I thought I was dealing with my plight quite well, but just recently I've had some mourning sessions concerning my body. I begin by mourning being without one breast, and then I move on to my half a femur that is gone—I had a hip replaced seven years ago. Add to that the pictures of women you see on TV and in magazines. This morning our guest minister did a quick summary of each of the Ten Commandments, and I heard the command "Do not covet. . ." in a very different way. He mentioned the regular things that we covet, like material things and such, but I thought of how easily it could be for me to begin coveting what others have, such as a healthy body. It was a good reminder for me to be thankful for what I have had and what I continue to be blessed with.

I'm reading a book about Afghanistan right now which is a great reminder of the great blessings I have received just because I was born in the United States. Not only am I thankful for comfortable living but also for wonderful doctors, technicians, and hospitals that can care for our illnesses. I wanted to join my grandsons as they sang our prayer at noon today. They called it the "Hoefie" prayer. (They learned this prayer at the Vande Hoef's). It goes like this—"God our Father, God our Father, We thank Him, We thank Him, For our many blessings, For our many blessings. Amen. Amen." Out of the mouths of babes.

Monday, February 12, 2007 9:33 a.m.

Yesterday was an amazing day. First of all, a friend of mine from church told me that they were discussing my situation at home and their five-year-old daughter (Bev Altena, you would know who this is) piped up and said, "What's wrong with my poor singin' Cella?" As I said yesterday, "Out of the mouths of babes!" Then Mindy, Sou, and the boys delivered a wonderfully delightful package from the library staff at Dordt. They knew my likes. Sherri, you don't have to worry about my wanting chocolate anymore. In fact, I should probably share some, but you have to come to Sanborn to get a taste. Thank you, ladies, for that great pick-me-upper. A little later Janie Van Dyke stopped over with some good home cooking from her mother and another big surprise—her niece Jessica Looman, who has and continues to struggle with cancer, sent Janie to deliver the cutest hat and headbands. (Jessica, you can't imagine how I felt. Here you are struggling with your own health, and you took time to remember me.) God continues to bless me. Ed, you were right, (see guest book entry) the love and support of the Christian community abounds, but it really kicks in during "helpless" situations. As you can see, we are "tasting" it in bigger and bolder ways. We continue to be blessed with delicious meals, cards, and encouragement through the CaringBridge site. You have all helped to make this experience a time to see God's love in action.

Soon I will leave to see Dr. Krie (the oncologist) and Dr. Stelzer (the surgeon). I will post what we find out later this afternoon. After my appointments I hope to go to visit my dad who is hospitalized in the Rock Valley hospital with lung problems. We hope and pray the treatments will help him recover soon.

Monday, February 12, 2007 7:34 p.m.

Life is like a roller coaster. How many times have you heard that? We've experienced this in our life. Since the last doctor's visit we felt as if we were going up the hill, but today our ride dove down into the valley. We were not prepared for what Dr. Krie told us today, and actually she was very surprised by the report too. The pathology report came back that the spot on my lung is cancer. If you know me, you know that I can't take amusement rides—they make me sick. That is exactly how I felt when Dr. Krie gave us the news. All I could think of was NO! NO! NO! Not me! I have so much I want to do yet. Lord, you have work for me to do. I thought of my grandchildren—I want to see them sing in the choir; I want to see them play the violin (my dream for at least one of my grandchildren); I want to see them play soccer and basketball. And will I? I don't know. The doctor said that only God knows. She said that the cancer has already determined where it will go, and now all we can do is do our best to fight against it.

I will have a brain scan yet this week and a port put in next Monday. Because a side effect of the chemo is bleeding, all my incisions must be completely healed before I can begin treatments. She is assuming, if all goes well, that I will begin treatments in five weeks. She's fairly sure of the treatment she will prescribe, but there are some details to work out. One of the details is making sure our insurance company will pay for one of the drugs which is unbelievably costly.

As I was riding home today (yes, we did the Bosma thing and each had our vehicle in Sioux Center), I thought about a little story that Megan told me this week. Here it is: Amira came home from school this week and said, "I've been shot." Surprised, Megan said, "What?" "I've been shot in the heart with a bow and arrow," exclaimed Amira. "Love shot me!"

As I was struggling to think of scripture that could help me adjust to this new diagnosis, Amira's story reminded me of II Thessalonians 2:16: "May our Lord Jesus Christ himself and God our Father, who loved us and by his grace gave us eternal encouragement and good hope, encourage your hearts and strengthen you in every good deed and word." I felt as if I was smitten with God's arrow of love and I know that feeling will continue as we ride the roller coaster. So many of you have assured me that you will help us as we have our ups and downs. We thank you for that. I know that even through hard times, or should I say, especially during hard times ". . . that neither death nor life, neither angels nor demons, neither the present nor the future, nor any powers, neither height nor depth, nor anything else in all creation, will be able to separate us from the love of God that is in Christ Jesus our Lord" (Romans 8:38-39). "No, in all these things we are more than conquerors through him who loved us" (Romans 8:37).

Please continue to pray with us.

Tuesday, February 13, 2007 7:58 a.m.

Good Morning,

And what a good morning it was for me this morning! Jerry had been up for hours moving snow, so I was surprised when he walked into the bedroom but even more surprised when he had a bunch of people with him. Megan's coworkers at De Vos Children's Hospital began a collection three weeks ago so that she and Mike and the kids could come home. I thought I was dreaming at first. I've had other not so pleasant dreams lately (I think it is the pain medication) so this seemed like the dream of all dreams! It was true; there stood Mike, Megan, Amira, and Nico! When you get down, God does send blessings to renew your spirit. Thank you from the bottom of our hearts to all of Megan's friends at work for making this possible. We are still speechless at your generosity.

Today Mindy and I were planning to choose a wig so now Megan can go with us. My doctor has a wonderful service that provides a wig for each of her patients. I can choose the color and style and then they order it especially designed for me. Another little blessing. I'll write more later. I hope you have as wonderful a day as I plan to have. In Him.

Wednesday, February 14, 2007 8:27 a.m.

Good Morning. The sun is shining and the snow is glistening and it is Valentine's Day.

Wow! What a difference a few extra people in the house makes—no time to dwell on sad thoughts and there is lots of joy and laughter. (Josh came home yesterday too. He had been sledding in the Big Horns.) I spent the day with the girls and Nico. We had a wonderful time. We began by visiting my dad in the hospital, going out for a wonderful and delicious lunch, and then we did some shopping. It reminded me of the days when the girls were still at home (except for visiting dad in the hospital). The girls (and me too) giggled about many remembrances from the past. We would ride by something and say, "Remember when . . ." and bust into laughter." Ah, memories—build them; they are good things to come back to during reflective times in your life. Mike's parents came for supper last night; friends stopped, so our day passed quickly.

After the last light was shut off last night and the house was quiet, I did have time to reflect. When I read Sandi's entry this morning, it re-minded me of what I read last night. The book, given to me by a friend, is called *A Reason for Hope* and that is the topic of the book. The reminders I read last night talked about the triggers of hope:

- being treated by doctors who are committed to finding the best treatments
- being surrounded by hopeful people (family and friends)
- reading great books, including the Bible, to boost my hope

The book reminded me that the living God is my source of hope. He is helping me receive this last piece of news, "not as if it is the last edition, but as if it is one piece of information afloat on a river of facts flowing into a hopeful future." My prayer today is—ground my hope in the reality of Your profound and enduring love for me and Your desire for my well-being. Hebrews 2:13 says this: "And again, 'I will put my trust in Him.' And again he says, 'Here am I . . . .'"

Happy Valentine's Day! Be sure to take time to express your love to those you love and to those who maybe aren't so lovable but need you.

Thursday, February 15, 2007 7:39 a.m.

As I was reading and reflecting this morning, I came upon the well-known verses from Proverbs: "Trust in the LORD with all your heart and lean not on your own understanding; in all your ways acknowledge him, and he will make your paths straight." I think that is emerging as one of the battles right now. It's been a while since I have had to really trust. Oh, I trust each and every day, but it's not the same now. Each and every day now is different. My routine is gone. I'm not sure from day to day what is going to happen. Just when I think, "No more doctor appointments for awhile," one is scheduled. Just when I think I know what is happening, I realize I don't.

I read a devotional that helped me understand and take comfort in Proverbs 3:5-6. It said life is like a bike ride, a tandem bike. Sometimes we act like we are in the driver's position and we steer and guide and decide, but when we let go and let God do the steering, life takes on a whole new perspective. The devotional suggested that when we think we know the way, life is pretty predictable (something I rather like). We take the shortest way between two points. But when God is leading, He takes us to delightful long cuts, up mountains, through rocky places, and at breakneck speeds. Sometimes it feels as if all we can do is to hang on. When the path becomes difficult and it looks crazy to us, God says, "Pedal." When we aren't sure what is ahead and we hold our anxious breath, that's when we learn to trust. That's when we realize that God knows the "bike secrets." He knows how to bend to make the sharp corners, how to jump to miss the rocks, when to speed up and when to slow down.

As I learn to trust, I hope I'll be able to enjoy the adventure. I'll meet new people, become more knowledgeable, become more empathetic, and I hope, find life even more exciting. God says, "Come along and trust me." I'd love to know every detail—what lies beyond each bend and ridge, but God patiently says, "Just trust me."

I'm working on that. Please pray that I can find that trust each and every day. I pray I can let God steer and I can pedal like mad. Again, thank you so much for your prayers, concerns, care, and even the surprises that you have brought my way. I love all of you!

By the way, if you want to see some cute kids, be sure to check my photo page.

Thursday, February 15, 2007 8:53 a.m.

Can you add one more thing to your prayer list? I just got a call that Josh cut the tip of his finger off at work. Jerry just left for the hospital and

I'll leave soon. Thanks.

Thursday, February 15, 2007 12:26 p.m.

Amazingly we are already back from Josh's surgery. They found a surgeon in Spencer who could take him immediately so the ambulance brought him there. Jerry and I got to the hospital just as the surgeon was finishing the last stitches. We could take him home with us, and he is now resting. I have an appointment to keep so I'll keep you posted a little later. Wow! Life keeps adding new twists.

Friday, February 16, 2007 7:46 a.m.

Good Morning,

First of all, I want to thank all of you for continuing to remember me in many ways. Each day I open either my guest book, my e-mail, or my snail mail and I am amazed at who I am getting encouragement from. I would love to mention names, but I'm sure I would leave someone out. Some encouragement comes from dear friends that I have lots of contact with, but I've been encouraged also by some of you whom I haven't seen in a long time. I have loved hearing from far-away and near nephews, nieces, students I taught in elementary school, my present and past college students, high school friends, colleagues, teachers I have taught with or had contact with, old friends, new friends, friends of our children, and relatives. Today again I opened greetings that were very encouraging. Thanks.

Yesterday again added to the roller coaster ride. Even though Josh's finger was quite easily "fixed," it was an emotional event for me (and for Josh). When I heard the news, my first thought was—not one more thing, I don't want another thing. But as usual God's grace set in. It was one more opportunity for me to pedal from the back seat and let God steer from the front. (If you don't understand this, read yesterday's journal.)

Josh seemed to breeze through the surgery and felt good until the pain block ran out. It was late into the evening when the pain began and it didn't take long for us to realize he would never sleep with all that pain. We called the doctor who told us to take Josh to the emergency room for a shot for the pain. Jerry took Josh to the Sheldon hospital and he received the shot. It was very effective and it allowed Josh to sleep well.

Remember yesterday I referred to the tandem bike. It was interesting that this morning I read another devotional referencing a bike. This example came from Joel Nederhood's book *The Forever People*. Jude

24-25 says, "To him who is able to keep you from falling . . . be glory, majesty, power, and authority. . . . " Dr. Nederhood says, "God is like a father who runs beside his little child's two-wheeler when she first learns to ride, keeping up with her, speaking a few instructions, always ready with His hand to steady the bike—God guards us from falling that way." Whether it be a physical fall or an emotional fall, God does a superior job of holding us in His hand. We felt that hand yesterday. Each day we are thankful for the Spirit of God that works in our hearts and gives us courage to face each new day. Each day we experience His glory, majesty, power, and authority.

Our prayer for today is: Please, O loving God, keep me from falling today. Help us to pedal from behind and let you do the steering. I pray in Jesus' name, who has given us the Spirit of perseverance. Amen.

Saturday, February 17, 2007 9:01 a.m.

Yesterday was full of good news—My dad was released from the hospital; Marcia, my twin sister who just began her chemo treatments, was feeling better; Josh was given stronger pain medication so he felt much relief; I had my site drained one more time. It looks as if the site is almost finished draining which is really good news because I have to finish receiving pokes into my skin so we can set a chemo date. I will have my port put in on Monday. They are assuming that this incision will be healed in four weeks.

Last night we attended a birthday party of a wonderful friend. It was great to be surrounded by friends I hadn't seen in a while. Through conversations I had I was reminded of the necessity of taking one day at a time. We found this advice important when we were dealing with Josh's head injury. When we looked too far ahead we got discouraged. I'm not sure I'm theologically correct on this but I've come to realize that, in my experiences, God has always given us grace for the day. When I look into the future I begin to fabricate and I see what could be, not what is. God gives me grace for what I'm experiencing, not grace for what I imagine could happen. Sometimes we watch others go through trials and we say, "How can they handle . . . ?" They've received God's grace and that's what's helping them cope. So my prayer for today comes from Paul in II Corinthians 12:9: "My grace is sufficient for you, for my power is made perfect in weakness." My Bible commentary said Paul was a very self-sufficient person, so his thorn must have been difficult for him. The affliction kept Paul humble, reminded him of his need for constant contact with God, and benefited those around him as they saw God's work in his life. If my illness can in some small way accomplish this, praise God. Please help me pray to be able to keep my eyes on God for His day-to-day grace.

Thanks for the bold prayers, for your encouragement, and for the fun stories that you tell through your entries. I love hearing from you. Peace.

Sunday, February 18, 2007 8:53 a.m.

What a beautiful morning. The sun is shining brightly, the snow is glistening, and the temperature promises to be warmer. And it's Sunday!

At my last doctor's appointment with Dr. Krie, she encouraged me to think about the things I have always wanted to do but didn't take the time for. Over the past few years I've wanted to take my grandsons sledding but there never seemed to be enough snow on days we could go. Well, yesterday that wish came true, only it was even more blessed because we got to go sledding with just about everyone in the family. The Prins family invited our church members to their hill. So everyone but Josh and Jerry trekked through the nearly knee-deep snow to the hill. What fun! The kids squealed with delight as they scooted down the hill. It was fun to watch (and sled too) as the kids' paths often crossed each other and they toppled over in the snow. (Look for pictures later today.) It was great fun to enjoy this with the family. Being out in the cold, crisp air and plowing through the snow was exhilarating! Isn't it too bad that a sudden diagnosis has to be the cause for taking time out to enjoy simple things?

This morning I was reading another devotional by Joel Nederhood, *This Splendid Journey*. It was based on Psalm 55 which talks about the troubles of David. This Psalm contains one of my favorite verses: "Cast your cares on the LORD . . ." (vs. 22). The Hebrew word for care here is only used once in the Bible. It means care in its broadest and widest sense. When we cast our cares upon God, He will sustain us. "This is the Holy Spirit's word sent our way by the God who suffered more than any of us ever will." If you have cares, I hope you too can give them over to our comforting and sustaining Lord. I pray that each of you who reads this can enjoy this day, praising God for His sustaining love and care.

Have a good day.

Monday, February 19, 2007 8:08 a.m.

Good Morning,

In just a few minutes I'm leaving for the hospital so Dr. Stelzer can put a port in my chest. No more pricks for me! From now on all blood draws and injections, including chemo, will be through the port. I have needle phobia, so the past month has been stressful for me. I'm glad the port will alleviate any more needle pokes in my arms.

Our minister Pastor Greg Dyk introduced the morning service yesterday by reminding us of the beauty of the glistening snow. He said that just as the sun makes the snow glisten, so should we glisten because of the Son. Since then I've been trying to think of ways that I can glisten for Him, even as I enter the hospital today and have another procedure. I hope those who work on me will see my love for God. How will you glisten today?

Monday, February 19, 2007 9:14 p.m.

We have been very busy and have had much fun this last week. I've tried very hard to be content being a part of things via phone calls from Michigan . . . , but I won't lie that it's been much better being here. We tried to capture some of the fun we've had the last couple of days through the pictures we posted . . . sledding, eating chocolate, birthday parties, grandparents piled with grandkids, and my favorite moment from last week—wig shopping. We obviously wouldn't prefer to have to go through that, but since we must, we decided to have fun and boy did we. When we came out of the "salon," the woman at the cash register commented that she wished she could have been part of the party. We giggled lots and discovered that mom looks beautiful as brunette, blonde, or grey. We got the cutest wig out there. Talk about grace for the moments. We've been blessed through the moments and by all of you. The guest book on this site, the 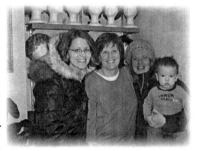 cards in the mail, the meals for my parents and Josh, my coworkers helping me fly back to Michigan, and all the other acts of kindness that have been shown to us—thank you hardly seems enough. From the bottom of our hearts, we do thank you and praise God for all of you.

About today's events—mom had her port placed late this morning. It hurt more than the nurses prepared her for. I think she needed a child-life specialist with the "NO Surprises" motto to prepare her.

Mike and Amira are safely back in Michigan; Nico and I are looking forward to one more week with Mom and the rest of our family.

I'm eagerly anticipating the grace and memories that I'm confident we'll continue to experience throughout the moments of this coming week. Megan

Tuesday, February 20, 2007 9:43 a.m.

Even though I really dislike winter, I do love to look out and see the beauty of the season. The whiteness of the landscape is a clear reminder to me of the amazing way our lives are made white through Jesus Christ. But I am looking forward to spring—it reminds me of Christ too. The signs of new life are a great reminder of the new life we have in Him. As Megan said, I was not prepared for the discomfort of the port, but today most of the pain is gone and I feel awake. I pretty much slept the day away yesterday. Today is going to be a lazy day. I'm planning to do some things for school during the day and then attend Kobi's preschool program this evening. I, like any grandma, am very excited to see him in his first program. Talk to you later.

Wednesday, February 21, 2007 7:42 a.m.

To my dear friends,

Yesterday was one of those days—one of those long roller coaster rides. It started the minute I got in the shower and seemed to go on until I closed my eyes. As in real life, I get off the ride exhausted and harried— that's how I felt at the end of the day. As I reflected on the day and tried to identify what was driving the anxiety, I couldn't put my finger on one thing but I do believe that a couple of really fun things triggered the feeling. Isn't that odd? Megan and I picked out a frame for our family picture 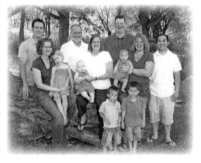 yesterday. My humanness gave in to thoughts of how many more would we take. We also watched Kobi in his first-ever school program. It was wonderful. He was so cute, sang every word, and did every action. To a grandma, he was the best child on the stage. But again thoughts of how many programs will I see set in.

Humanness; it's the pits.

This morning I picked up a devotional and the title was "Are You Afraid?" (Of course I am, you idiot.) It gave the account from Luke 8:22-25 where the disciples were afraid of being dumped into the sea because of the storm. After Jesus quieted the storm he asked them, "Where is your faith?" The disciples had seen Jesus perform miracle after miracle, yet they experienced fear. Feeling fearful is human. Yet we must all learn the lesson that the disciples learned: Jesus was in the boat with them. Just as He was there for them, He is here for us too. None of us are alone. My voyage, like yours, continues, but the waters can remain calm if we fix our eyes on Jesus.

Pastor Rod Gorter called yesterday and the words that he spoke and the verses he gave me helped calm the waters. He reminded me of Isaiah 41:13: "For I am the Lord, your God, who takes hold of your right hand and says to you, Do not fear; I will help you."

I'm praying: Bring, I pray, calm to the raging storms in my life. I am afraid of the cancer; I'm afraid of the future, but I am not afraid of You. Help me place my trust in You and You alone. I offer this humble prayer in the name of the Great Physician, Jesus Christ. Amen.

Thursday, February 22, 2007 7:46 a.m.

Recently many of you have reminded me that none of us know what that future holds. I may have been diagnosed with cancer (I don't want to sound morbid), but my time on earth may be longer than any one of you reading this entry. None of us know the number of our days. I was doubly reminded of this today when I heard of the deaths of two young people who were very close to the age of our son Joshua. How my heart breaks for the Lange and Dykstra families. What a shock it must have been to learn of their children's deaths. I hope they, like me, find comfort in Psalm 90 and 91. I hope you can find time to read them too. In Psalm 90 Moses reminds us: "Teach us to number our days aright, that we many gain a heart of wisdom." What a reminder that life is short and that we must use the time we have wisely.

On one of his videos, Harry Wong, a well-known educator with an unfortunate name, asks his students this question, "What will you do today to make this world a better place?" I like to challenge my students to ask themselves these questions, "What will you do today to enhance God's kingdom? How will you show, today, that God is the Lord of your life?" I have to ask myself these questions too—constantly. Megan has often reminded me of that while she has been home; she wants to know in the midst of all the love we are receiving, what we are going to do to show God's love to someone else? We don't ask ourselves these questions to work ourselves into the good graces of God, but I hope to live out the love we have for Him. And for the sheer fact that it feels good to help make this world a better place and to think of others rather than ourselves. The days of the two young people have been numbered. I hope their families can find comfort in the first two verses of Psalm 91: "He who dwells in the shelter of the Most High will rest in the shadow of the Almighty. I will say of the Lord, 'He is my refuge and my fortress, my God, in whom I trust.'" This is a comfort for all of us.

Please join me in praying for these families.

A little bit about my health. Thanks to lots of encouragement, I felt emotionally much stronger yesterday. I was again astonished by the number of people who remembered me—former students, past colleagues, old friends, cousins—you know who you are. Each and every one of you inspired me with your words and letters of encouragement. I am grateful for all of you. As far as my physical health, the port site is feeling much better. The swelling is going down and I don't feel as if I'm being pulled to the ground when I bend over. My surgical site is healing very nicely. I've sworn off razors to avoid any cuts. Don't worry, I'm not joining the Dutch women; I'll find other methods for shaving, for as long as I have to anyway. There will be some blessings to having no hair (notice how happy my smiley face is without hair.) As soon as my incisions heal, I'll be able to begin treatments. I'll find out about treatments on March 2. My right arm is beginning to feel more normal although I still have tingling and tightness. Originally I was told that the tingling could last forever, so I am extremely happy to feel the healing taking place. My brain scan is scheduled for next Tuesday.

I've heard from many of you that you are joining us in prayer, not only individuals but school staffs and many classes. How can I say thanks? I'm not sure how. I will never be able to thank you enough, but be assured that my family and I are forever grateful.

Tuesday, February 27, 2007 7:02 a.m.

Good Morning,

I can't believe it has been so long since I wrote in my journal. My life was on the fast pace the past few days. On Friday morning I joined the education department on a curriculum retreat on Friday and Saturday. It was much fun to think about school things again and to enjoy fellowship with my colleagues.

When my friends left for home, I stayed in Sioux Falls. My family came up and we enjoyed a couple of fun days in a hotel. Megan and Nico were supposed to fly out Sunday morning and we thought we should be close to the airport in case driving would be difficult because of the weather. Being in Sioux Falls didn't help; her plane was canceled and she wasn't able to get on a plane until Monday morning. It was wonderful to have her here, but I know it was time for her to get back to her own family and work. Amira was missing her terribly and I think Mike was too. Child-life specialist at De Vos, we're giving her back to you. Please take good care of her! Thanks much for the kindness and friendship you have lavished on her the past few weeks. You've been a blessing!

I was reminded the past weekend of Proverbs 17:22: "A cheerful heart is good medicine, but a crushed spirit dries up the bones." There have been some days when it has been difficult to have a cheerful spirit. Sometimes I look too far ahead toward things I do not know and may not be reality. I'm not naive enough to think that laughter can heal me, but I do know that laughter is good medicine. Cancer isn't funny but we can find laughter in the midst of the cancer. A book I read said that sometime you have to look for it and sometime you have to create it, but that wasn't the case for me this weekend. Enjoying friends, watching my grandchildren swim, tromping through the snow, maybe didn't produce belly laughs, but they sure brought smiles and much pleasure.

I hope that all of you who read this will find something to smile about today, and maybe you'll be fortunate to even have a good belly laugh. I'd like to hear about them!

Yesterday the doctor checked my surgical sites and said both were healing very nicely. I've been worried about the pain in the port site but he said I bruised more than usual and that was causing the pain. He felt that with regular chemo, I would be able to begin treatments as early as next week, but since mine has the side effects of bleeding, it may take a little longer. This was the questionable drug for which we were waiting approval, and we heard this weekend that it was approved. We were very thrilled and thankful for this news. I'm leaving in a short while for the brain scan. It's not supposed to be a big deal and they aren't really looking to see any cancer there. The test is for surety and developing a baseline. Please pray that their assumptions turn out to be true.

Again, thanks for all the ways you continue to encourage me. I'll be on the site more this week. I hope you all enjoy your day.

Tuesday, February 27, 2007 12:17 p.m.

A quick update from this morning. The brain scan went well. It was quick and easy. After the scan I stopped in to see Dr. J. and from the symptoms I explained, he is quite sure that I came down with food poisoning this weekend. I'm miserable from the food poisoning but I am glad I didn't infect the whole family. More later.

Tuesday, February 27, 2007 6:35 p.m.

Dear friends and family,

Thanks much for the many meaningful journal entries over the past few weeks. I enjoy every one of them. I wish I could comment on each of them, but that not being possible, I've decided to pick a few out today. Some of you give me deep content to think about; some of you have made me laugh. Deb, I remember those bridges too. My project-based education wasn't always the delight of the parents, but we surely learned a lot! (How could I ever forget Kyle and Sonya? I have fond memories of them.) Shelley, your reminder that the Spirit intercedes was very comforting. Kim, I want you to know that I'm proud to be your cousin and glad to share some of the same characteristics, even if others don't appreciate them. Rick, your reminder to hold on to the blessings prayed for by the many who are lifting me up in prayer has strengthened me. Darlene, hearing that you are using my journal with your students has again humbled me. I remember using the prayer board in my classrooms, using it to help my students remember to pray for people with special needs, and now I feel blessed to have children and teachers in schools praying for me. For all of this, I say thanks. Thanks from the bottom of my heart. Thanks for the encouragement. I especially needed it today (more on that later.) If I didn't mention you, it wasn't because I overlooked your message. Every message lifts my heart!

Wednesday, February 28, 2007 7:37 a.m.

Good Morning,

Be still. How many ways can you say it: Be quiet, don't move, lie still, hang in there for a minute, don't breathe, hold it right there. I can't count the variety of ways I've been asked not to move over the past month. I'm not sure why but this morning as I was once again asked to lie still, I was overcome with emotion. I'm not always sure what triggers my emotions, but these words are starting to "bring it on." I felt sorry for the technicians as they tried to assure me that it would be an easy test. I told them I wasn't scared of it. They offered me tissues, patted my hands, and offered words of encouragement. I hated making them feel uncomfortable, but I couldn't seem to help what was happening. I tried to stuff the tears back to their proper place with very little success. What do you do with a woman through whom you are about to run a tube, who is not supposed to move, and you see the tears sneak out of the corner of the eyes and drop on the blanket cradling her head? What do you do as you watch her bite her lip so the sobs won't disturb the test? Not much more than they did, I guess. I wasn't scared of the test; I'm not even terribly worried about the results, so I'm not sure why the emotions today. But I do know that as I waited for the completion of the test, I had time to reflect on those all too familiar words, "Be still." "Be still, and know that I am God." Psalm 46:10 is what ran through my mind as my head was traveling back and forth through the tunnel. He is God! He is my strength, my strong tower, my fortress, my Maker. He continues to remind me with every "be still" that He wants me to fall into his loving arms and trust His care for me. When I become scared, I need to remember that God is in control, and He will never leave me nor forsake me. All I need to do is "Be still, and know . . . ."

Throughout the night, I continued to feel the effects of the food poisoning. My stomach still lurched and growled, my chest still felt tight and congested and my cough hacky, but this morning I feel a lot of relief. The doctor said the symptoms shouldn't last past Thursday. And wouldn't you know it, I thought I had finished going to my last doctor's appointment when something else happened. I haven't eaten much since noon on Sunday so last night when I smelled the delicious chicken casserole that someone had brought in to us, I couldn't help eating a little dish of it. I thought it might be a little heavy for a stomach that had no food, but I had to try it. Well, after about three bites, it wasn't my stomach that I was worried about. I felt myself biting on a hard object. I pulled the object out of my mouth and discovered a cap from one of my teeth. I'll need to call both Dr. Krie and my dentist today. Dr. Krie said I shouldn't have any dental work done close to my treatments because of the side effect of bleeding. One more trip to a doctor! Take care!

March/April 2007

Thursday, March 1, 2007 10:04 a.m.

My Internet has been down. What a bother.

Yesterday a cousin of mine, Judy Vanden Bosch, sent me a song that again reminded me of God's faithfulness. It is titled "He's Always Been Faithful" and it is sung by Sara Groves.

Here are the lyrics:

Great is thy faithfulness, Lord, unto me

Morning by morning I wake up to find
The power and comfort of God's hand in mine
Season by season I watch Him, amazed
In awe of the mystery of His perfect ways
All I have need of, His hand will provide

He's always been faithful to me.
I can't remember a trial or a pain
He did not recycle to bring me gain
I can't remember one single regret
In serving God only, and trusting His hand
All I have need of, His hand will provide
He's always been faithful to me.

This is my anthem, this is my song
The theme of the stories I've heard for so long
God has been faithful, He will be again
His loving compassion, it knows no end
All I have need of, His hand will provide
He's always been faithful, He's always been faithful
He's always been faithful to me.

The music to this song is very soothing and comforting. The tune was new to me, but it did incorporate one small musical line from the song we all know: "Great is Thy Faithfulness." I love the old with the new. But it wasn't the tune that drew me into the song. It was the lyrics. As I read through them, I thought of all the ways I had seen God's faithfulness work in my own life.

29

Today I reflected on the first verse. It reminded me of my confidence that every single day, God will send the sun to open up the day. We may not always see it, like today, but I know it's up there—for sure! Each fall I know that the leaves are going to drop from the trees; I know that we are going to have cold temperatures in the winter and warmer temps in the summer. This never fails. Sometimes things change a bit, but they never fail. Those are His perfect ways. I've seen God's perfect ways in things other than nature too. I think of how God guided our son-in-law Souvanna and his family from the country of Laos to the United States. He took them through rice paddies as their young children sucked on chicken bones to keep them from crying so they wouldn't be found by the army that was patrolling the area. God directed their path to Sioux Center, Iowa, where he grew up to know the Lord and has been used to influence the lives of many young people. Not only am I thankful for that, but I'm thankful that we have been given Sou. I'm thankful for what he adds to our family, for how he complements Mindy, and for the three beautiful children they share with us. I'm amazed at His perfect ways—that's how Sou became part of our family. It's one of the things that assures me of God's faithfulness.

I spent most of yesterday trying to find the energy to do something. I wasn't too successful. I'm still struggling with the results of the food poisoning. Although the stomach cramps have somewhat subsided, I'm still having a difficult time eating. My ears and throat still hurt and my chest still feels full. My voice is still raspy but not too raspy for Amira to recognize it. I did get the crown put back on my tooth today. I'm thankful for a great dentist who was willing to fit me into his schedule and recap my tooth.

I'm feeling much better today. It looks as if it is going to be a stay-in day today. I'm hoping we'll be able to get to the doctor tomorrow, but we'll have to wait and see what the weather does.

Friday, March 2, 2007 7:13 a.m.

Oh what a beautiful white morning! No, I haven't lost my mind. Most of you who know me, know my dislike for winter. I'm ready for warm weather and flowers. But we don't always have to like everything to see how it can bring joy to someone else. Jerry loves winter and he loves snow. He has had to give up much the past month. He has taken time off work, sat in the hospital, served meals, washed the dishes, doted on me, and, last but not least, missed a snowmobile trip with his buddies. For the past 15 years, he has planned this trip so this was no easy thing to give up. Besides that, he hasn't even gotten to ride his snowmobile this winter. But he has never once complained. See why I love him? So, for all of you who dislike this last blast of snow, I hope it will help you to know that Jerry had the time of his life last night. He and Josh went out with some friends and hit all those nice soft piles of snow, and some that weren't so soft too. They spent a bit of time getting themselves unstuck. They came home like two little kids who'd been locked in a candy store.

"Rejoice in the Lord always. I will say it again: Rejoice!" (Philippians 4:4). Paul's lesson for us could be that our inner attitudes do not have to reflect our outer circumstances. Even if you don't like the snow, I hope it doesn't get in the way of your praising God for the wonderful day that He has provided. I praise God for the beauty of snow and the fun it can bring.

I'm feeling much better. I actually had ambition to work on school work yesterday. It felt good to accomplish something. My stomach is feeling better and so are my throat and ears. Night before last, I had such an earache that I asked Jerry to try a home remedy that my doctor told me about when my children were young. I laid my head sideways on the bar stool while Jerry poured warm olive oil into my ears. After each application we capped them with cotton balls. I also listened to Jerry and many of my other relatives who are always telling me to use Vicks. We laughed at our homeopathic concoctions. I stunk and looked ridiculous (with the little cotton balls poking out of my ears) but I felt a lot better in the morning so I guess it was worth it. I praise God for the many ways He heals us.

My doctor's appointment for today was postponed. The office called and rescheduled it for next Friday. I didn't think I could wait that long to hear about the brain scan or the treatment schedule so I called and got an appointment for next Monday. That means driving to Sioux Falls, but both Jerry and I felt it is worth it. We are both eager to see what lies ahead. I praise God for being able to reschedule.

Thanks for your continued e-mails, cards, and various ways you continue to encourage us. I've enjoyed your guest entries. I thank God for all of you. If you find time, I'd love to be smothered with prayers for patience until my Monday doctor's appointment. Amira could also use some prayers today. She's being x-rayed for a broken arm.

I praise God for you. "Rejoice in the Lord always. I will say it again: Rejoice!" (Philippians 4:4).

Friday, March 2, 2007 7:08 p.m.

I got a call from Megan while they were still in the x-ray department of the hospital. She said the x-rays confirmed that Amira had truly broken her arm—both bones. Amira, of course, had the best care with her mom and her child-life colleagues distracting and spoiling her. I could hear her in the background and she sounded pretty chipper. I bet none of you want to be in our family right now. I thought I'd let you know.

Saturday, March 3, 2007 8:04 a.m.

Oh what a beautiful day, literally!

Even though I would have rather gotten up this morning to flowers and green grass, I do have to admit that the winter wonder that is before me is magnificent. The trees are packed with snow and their limbs bent with all the weight. Our white poles sparkle as the sun's rays shine upon them and I have to admit that winter is a gift from God, not one I always appreciate but one that shows us God as a magnificent creator. Did you see all the creations in the snow that the wind conjured up? So many different shapes and sizes.

They reminded me of you. Just as I see beauty and variety as I look out the window, so I see beauty and variety when I think of all of you. So many people and many blessings. (Okay, so I'm crying again.) You all bless me in many ways. Yesterday I snooped on the M&Ms and peanuts that Jaleesa and Sara brought over. Okay, so they probably didn't bless my hips but they sure did a lot for cabin fever. My neighbor Phyllis blessed me by letting me cry on her shoulder. We are still eating the delicious soup that Marilyn brought over. It was one of many meals that people graciously made for us. Aunt Nance blessed me with a lovely e-mail. Gail made me laugh and ponder. Kim and Jill reminded me of their love for my family. Carol and Carrie had me reflecting on the value of old and deep friendships. Shar gave me the reminder of the joy of the telephone (okay, everybody in the family, quit smiling!). My dean Sherri blessed me by letting me know that she never quits caring and my dear friend Pat showed me that she continues to support me with her loving and caring advice. I can't forget the visit with which Nate and Cath blessed me or the conversation I had with Lorna in the grocery store. My mom's parting remark was that she is praying for me, one gift I know that I have received from many of you. And the list could go on. Your acts of kindness have not gone unnoticed, even if I haven't mentioned it.

God has equipped each of you with special gifts and talents to be used for His glory. You have used them to minister to me and often just when I've needed them the most. Thank you much for being willing to give of your time and sharing your gifts with me. I couldn't be where I am emotionally without you. You are able to make all grace abound to me, so that in all things and at all times, having all that I need, I will abound in every good work. You faithfully provide. (Scripture reference II Corinthians 9:8). I know that you are glorifying God. Praise You.

Sunday, March 4, 2007 6:45 a.m.

Hello friends—Happy Sunday,

Though I don't like winter, the snowstorm we had showed the awesome power of God. After the terrible winds we experienced, we feel our weakness all the more. It's a great reminder of the importance of taking advantage of all the ways that are available to help us deepen our relationship with God, one of them being that we are able to attend church. What a blessing and one we sometimes forget. We have many opportunities to ground ourselves in God's Word but often feel too busy to take the time for them. Sometimes it takes a jolt to get us to recognize them. Storms have the potential to do that. I hope you sense God's power as I do.

This morning I got up and can finally say that I think most of the symptoms of the food poisoning are gone. All that's left is a slightly stuffed head and a hoarse voice. I'm glad that's over.

We're looking forward to a warmer day, melting snow, going to church, and having lunch with Mindy, Sou, and the boys. Today, among other things, our prayer is for a peaceful day as we anxiously await the news we will receive from Dr. Krie on Monday. I'm praying for positive news from the brain scan and the opportunity for treatments to begin soon. I hope you'll help us with that prayer. Thanks.

Monday, March 5, 2007 6:57 a.m.

We're on our way to Sioux Falls. Please pray that we will hear good news and that whatever news we receive, we will be surrounded by God's grace.

Monday, March 5, 2007 3:00 p.m.

After Dr. Krie's first piece of news this morning, I wanted to stand up and sing, "Praise God" at the top of my lungs, but instead I let it ring through my head. Dr. Krie assured us that the brain scan was clean. When she told us, we both heaved sighs of relief and then we dug into the other reason for the visit—the chemo treatments. Dr. Krie laid out the plan and just as she was finishing, I mentioned a perforation that I have had in my nasal membrane (I've had it for five years). She immediately became concerned, put me back on the examining table, and told me that she would have to reconsider the treatment plan. Because Avactin, the new drug that we were so excited about that was approved for me, causes bleeding, she is concerned that it could be a problem for me. She made an appointment for me to see an ear, nose, and throat doctor on Friday and we'll see from there. Just when we thought the road was straightening out, we find another bump. We are praying that the inside of my nose can be fixed quickly and that I can still take Avactin. We'll keep you posted.

I don't know how many prayers were offered for us today, but Jerry and I both commented on how, even though we were a bit nervous, we felt as if we were being carried on the wings of prayer. What a peaceful feeling. Both of us know that all of you have added to that feeling of peace. Your prayers (and other acts of kindness) have helped to lift this burden. We thank you for these prayers, and if we can be bold, we'd like to ask you to continue to pray for us. Please pray that my nose can be fixed quickly and that treatments can begin as soon as possible.

We humbly thank you.

Tuesday, March 6, 2007 7:40 a.m.

Good Morning, dear friends,

Last night I did something I haven't done in a long time—I went to a high school basketball game and actually watched the whole game from beginning to end. I loved it. It was exciting to be in a big crowd, cheering all together. Those young guys "ran the race." Up and down the floor, dribbling, screening, passing, shooting, defending. They worked hard from beginning to end. There were times disappointment registered on their faces. There were times you could see their faces radiate with pure joy. They worked hard and played as if their life depended on it. And in the end, after all that hard work, the victory was theirs. There was much cheering and yelling and lots of high fives. The coach raised his arms to form a V as he looked up at his wife (my friend, Sylvia) to say, "We won!" (Sylvia, I saw your happiness too.) What excitement!

Immediately after the game, we heard that my friends' (Janie and Libby) niece and sister had died. The excitement of the night turned to somberness. I felt pulled from polar ends. There was the excitement of being at a big game and the sadness of death. But then I had to tell myself that Jessica, too, ran the race. She persevered through obstacles that would have stopped the strongest. She may have lost the game here on earth, but she surely won the greatest battle of all and won the prize. My thoughts went back to the game and I thought about this momentous occasion for the team. They won the game but it seemed to me that they did more than just win a game. They showed us what life should be like—perseverance to the end and all the while with grace. I was impressed with the way they played the game. They played with a vengeance to win, but in all that play, they showed character. They played clean, worked hard, showed respect to the refs and other players, and took the win with grace. I didn't know Jessica well, but it seemed to me that's how she played her game too, with perseverance to the end, and all the while encouraging others in their "game."

The young men fought the good fight; they persevered until the end; they won the battle and so did Jessica.

I was very encouraged by the news of the clean brain scan yesterday, but to tell you the truth, the percentages that Dr. Krie quoted for those with metastasized cancer scared me. But my experiences last night encouraged me and taught me a lesson. I don't know what's going to happen in my life, but I do know that I can persevere just like that young team and Jessica, and in the end I hope, like Paul, I can say, "I have fought the good fight, I have finished the race, I have kept the faith" (II Timothy 4:7). The victory is mine.

Wednesday, March 7, 2007 6:53 a.m.

This is the Day!

This is the day that the Lord hath made, and I'm glad He made me (and you too). With each rising sun He is here by my side, He is more than a dream come true.

This is the day—the day I go back to the classroom. Today I will begin teaching one of my favorite classes and then next Monday, I'm hoping to pick up another one of my favorite classes. I'm very thankful. I'm looking forward to living on a schedule again (one that I hope doesn't include doctors:) and being in the classroom with my students, and being encouraged by my colleagues. If you can't tell, I'm very excited! Please pray that I can be effective in the classroom and that I can hold up both physically and emotionally. Ask my students; it doesn't take much for me to get emotional! Thanks for your continued support! I'm where I'm at emotionally because of all of you! Thank God too for a brand new day—a day that has been given to us so that we can show His glory. I can't wait!

Thursday, March 8, 2007 7:03 a.m.

Some thoughts:

To be truthful, I've had some moments these days when I wish all this would just pass, disappear, go away. Sometimes I do ask God (and I'm sorry to say, not so nicely) why all this is happening, and I beg Him to take it all away. Sometimes I think that this is all a bad dream, a nightmare actually, and that I'll wake up to a body that is cancer free. Sometimes I wish I could just reverse life and choose another "door." Isn't that what they do on "Let's Make a Deal"? But I can't. Life is where it's at and that's all there is to it.

But that's not really true—it's not all there is to it. There have been many blessings throughout this whole situation. One of the blessings was being able to get back in the classroom yesterday with that fresh excitement that comes with a new assignment. I felt nervous—that almost heady feeling; the adrenalin pulsated through me. It felt good to be in a learning environment once again, a learning environment that has to do with education and not medicine. It truly fits me better. Again today I received encouraging posts on the CaringBridge site, cards that were thoughtful, songs that inspired me, conversations that lifted my spirit, hugs (some imaginary) that squeezed me, and some big beautiful daisies that brightened my office. Two days ago, two students came and pampered me with a facial and yesterday three students took me out for lunch. So many of you have taken precious time to pray for me. I have felt loved very much.

One of the things this experience has shown me is that God's people truly do care. They understand what it means to provide support. When I think of your care, I can't help but think of the care my Savior has for me. He is the ultimate caretaker, the one who supplies my every need. I need that supply in a big way right now, and it is being supplied by Him through you. I can't imagine going through this without you. I feel that I am the recipient of Peter's instructions: "Each one should use whatever gift he has received to serve others, faithfully administering God's grace in its various forms . . . . If anyone serves, he should do it with the strength God provides, so that in all things God may be praised through Jesus Christ. To him be the glory and the power forever and ever. Amen" (I Peter 4:10, 11b).

My prayer is that through this all, the world may see that you and I are glorifying God and bringing Him honor and glory.

Friday, March 9, 2007 10:26 a.m.

Good Morning,

Isn't it a beautiful day? I was hoping to write in the journal this morning, but haven't found time. I'm heading to the ENT doctor in a few minutes. I'll post more about that later. I had another fantastic day in the classroom and am feeling blessed to be back at work. More later.

Saturday, March 10, 2007 7:45 a.m.

Good Morning,

Psalm 18:32-33 says this: "It is God who arms me with strength and makes my way perfect. He makes my feet like the feet of a deer; he enables me to stand on the heights." From day to day, I'm not sure how God is going to make my way perfect. It's especially difficult right now. I have a lot of questions: What will that perfection look like? How long will I have to wait to understand it? While I am waiting, I hang on to the promises of God—that He will give me strength to meet the challenges that come my way. I know that my problems are more than likely not going to be eliminated, but each day I do have the assurance that God will not leave me to walk by myself. That was evident again yesterday. I began the day somewhat anxious: would teaching go okay, would I have the energy to meet my students' needs, would I be able to concentrate on my work, what kind of news would I hear from the ENT doctor? All I had to do was trust, trust that He would enable me to stand on new heights.

Teaching went well, I accomplished a lot, and then I received yet another blessing. After examining me, the ENT doctor reported that the perforation in my septum was nothing to be concerned about. She said it shouldn't interfere with the chemo, and if a problem did arise, she could put a plug (yes, a plug!) in my nose. Thankfully it will be inside my nose so I won't have to worry about losing my job because of excessive body piercings. She is going to contact Dr. Krie and give the go-ahead for treatments. What a blessing! I am thankful for many things—for a good report on my nose, for a doctor who put together the treatment plan, and for an insurance company who okayed this treatment. Is this all part of the perfect way?

Mindy, Miles, and I spent the rest of the beautiful, warm afternoon doing a little shopping and, of course, celebrating with some treats. We shared a lot of laughs. What a blessing. By the way, Megan, because Mindy was with me, I never got lost once. My evening ended with an enjoyable supper with Jerry's family and then home to read my mail. Wow! I was blessed with many beautiful cards and notes again. Aunt Lucy sent me a very funny booklet, which Josh read to me from cover to cover; the Cary Christian Center's card reminded me that they are putting us in the arms of Jesus; Jill sent a hilarious picture from 1982, the year we won the Sheldon Slow Pitch softball tournament, (cute hairdos) and a long letter full of nostalgia; Uncle Tom and Aunt Laura gave me a devotional and bookmark of Heidelberg Catechism, Lord's Day 1, and Sylvia and Pam blessed me with encouraging words and the promise of prayer. I continue to be humbled and thankful for all your acts of kindness.

I thank my sovereign God for working on my path each day, for allowing things in my life for a greater purpose than I often understand. He is constantly in the practice of molding and making me more Christ-like and in this process, I know He will get me to where I need to be. Psalm 18:1: "I love you, O LORD, my strength."

Sunday, March 11, 2007 3:34 p.m.
Good Day,

What a different day today was than last week Sunday. The snow piles are going down and the air is warmer. Much to be thankful for. This morning we heard a wonderful sermon on Jesus' temptation in the wilderness. Our minister reminded us that each of us has our own wilderness, but like Jesus, we have a Father who is standing right beside us, ready to support us, keep us, hold us, make us strong, and He never lets go! I hope you too are feeling the loving hand of God as you travel your journey. We sang "Amazing Grace" in the service this morning. I didn't make it through the song. The words of this song, one of my favorites, reminded me once again of the amazing grace God gives to each one of us. I hope you are feeling God's amazing grace too.

We had a great lunch with Mindy, Sou, the boys, Josh, and our friends Nate and Cath. We hope to see my dad today and see how he is doing. Enjoy the spring-like weather.

Monday, March 12, 2007 7:47 a.m.
Last night we met with our Bible study group, one we've met with for many years, and yet again we felt the love of God through His people. Not only were they encouraging and supportive but they also presented us with a huge gift basket. What a blessing! After we got the emotions out of the way, we studied a lesson written by Rob Bell called "Rain." Rain, sometimes it comes down as soft gentle droplets, but other times we get plastered with hard pellets and it really hurts. Those are the times we cry out. The Psalms are full of verses that refer to crying.

Psalm 34:17: "Is anyone crying for help? God is listening, ready to rescue you." [MSG]

Psalm 55:17: "Evening, morning, and noon I cry out in distress and he hears my voice."

Psalm 72:12: "For he will rescue the poor who cry out and the afflicted who have no helper." [HCSB]

Sometimes we suppress our storms and we miss opportunities to cry to God and ask Him to comfort us or lead us through the storm. Rob Bell reminded us that God wants to hold us tight. It's in the stormy times we hear God say, "I love you!" I've heard that often the past two months. During these times I've felt Him hold me close and promise me that I'm going to make it.

Today I begin teaching one more class. It's another of my favorites. I'm looking forward to the contact with the students and the stimulation of teaching. Physically I'm feeling great right now, probably the best I've felt since January. I'm looking forward to the day and I hope you are too.

Tuesday, March 13, 2007 8:03 a.m.

Early this morning as I was thinking about the day and making plans to fill up each hour, I heard my husband snore and that led me to think about him. What a trooper he has been. Sometimes when we get hit with something, we become very self-absorbed. That's kind of where I've been. I've been consumed with doctors' appointments; I've focused on healing from surgery; I've thought about how God wants me to respond, but sometimes I've forgotten about Jerry. As I lay there thinking, I was struck by how much this has affected him too. He has had to miss days of work to accompany me on my medical visits. That not only put him behind in his work, but also affected his pay. He has had to answer thousands of questions, sometimes because I wasn't emotionally able to face them. He's made calls that I didn't want to make, picked up extra work at home, cooked, and cleaned; he's been super encouraging, not complaining about anything and has even given up his yearly snowmobile trips. He has always been strong, confident, positive and quick to step up to whatever is needed, and all the while he is scared and wondering about the future too. Yesterday one of his friends stopped by the house and told me what a great guy he was. I had to agree. Maybe that's what got me thinking about it this morning or maybe it was the snoring. I thank God for all of you but today I want to especially thank God for the gift of Jerry. Once again we see how God has showered us with His blessing. He's made Jerry strong and a great support for me. Ephesians

3:20 says this: "Now to him who is able to do immeasurably more than all we ask or imagine, according to his power that is at work within us, to him be glory in the church and in Christ Jesus . . . ." I thank God for the strength He has given Jerry.

I hope you have a good day. I don't teach today but I have meetings with students and our department. I am also looking forward to having lunch with a long-time friend Del Dykstra, with whom I taught at Sanborn Christian. I hope you will enjoy the warm temperatures as much as I will. Blessings to you as you travel through this day. May you find that immeasurable strength that God promises.

Wednesday, March 14, 2007 7:52 a.m.

A reflection on yesterday: Yesterday was a beautiful day. I woke to a sun-lit world and a hug from my husband (must have been an apology for the snoring). And that's the way the whole day went. As soon as I stepped out of my car on campus, I was greeted and warmly welcomed by a maintenance worker. As I walked up to the classroom building, I saw the door open and I was greeted by yet another staff member. Everywhere I went I felt warmly welcomed. Students were on campus for an interim. It was great to feel their hugs and hear their warm wishes. Colleagues continue to encourage me with smiles, hugs, and encouraging words. I got a hug from one of the deans of the college. Haven't gotten one from the president yet, but then again, I haven't seen him. Cards, e-mails, and CaringBridge comments give me hugs from a distance. And the biggest hug came from my friend Del whom I hadn't seen in a year.

As I was thinking about all these real and virtual hugs, I remembered the research I read recently on the importance of hugs. I can't remember how many hugs the research said that children need in order to produce their best work, but it was a lot. I'm thankful for all those hugs. But it also challenged me: Who am I going to hug today? Who will I find that needs that personal touch or "hello," or that smile? I'm going to be looking for someone and I hope you will too!

I Peter 1:22 reminds us: "Now that you have purified yourselves by obeying the truth so that you have sincere love for your brothers, love one another deeply, from the heart."

Thursday, March 15, 2007 1:45 a.m.

Acts 20:35 says "It is more blessed to give than to receive." That may be true, but I've also discovered for me personally, it is easier to give than to receive. That's how I feel tonight. A group of our friends and relatives got together and pooled money so that Jerry and I can take a vacation. It is a gracious act. We are excited and yet I feel anxious about going on a trip at the cost of others. Friends have told me to get over it and just enjoy. I'm working on it. I read a text from the Bible the other day (and I can't find it back) that said how rewarding it is for others to be able to help those who have struggles. I hope that all of you who have made this possible feel greatly rewarded.

A couple of weeks ago Dr. Krie encouraged us to plan a trip. She said it might be a while before we can do anything like this. We will be leaving this morning and will be gone until next Monday. The girls will probably post a few times while we are gone.

Dordt begins spring break tomorrow and since I don't teach on Thursday, it worked well for us to leave on Thursday. I'll begin treatments next Thursday, if all goes as planned, so we'll be home in time for me to get a few things in order before the long haul of treatments. I'm not sure if I've mentioned my treatment plan; if I have, sorry for the repetition. I will have one drug administered through my port once a week for three weeks and then have a week off. During that time, I will have another drug added every other week. So on the first and third week, I'll have two drugs put into the port. I will have three sessions of this and then I hope have another PET scan to see what is happening with my lung. I'm eager to get started on my treatments, but first of all I'm looking forward to a few days of rest and relaxation with Jerry.

There are many things I've learned already on this journey, but two that really stand out today are humility and gratitude. I'm humbled by the graciousness of many people—those of you who helped with the trip, but also those of you who continue to remember me in many ways, including praying. I'm grateful for all of you and thank you from the bottom of my heart for whatever you have done and continue to do for me and for my family. I'm working at receiving with grace.

With humility and gratitude.

Sunday, March 18, 2007 1:21 a.m.

I talked to mom tonight and they are having a wonderful time on their trip. They have gotten to relax and do some exciting different things that they don't get to do every day. We all want to thank everyone who made this much-needed trip possible for them. They have been able to enjoy each other's company and forget about everything that has been going on the last couple of months (as much as possible). We have all been amazed and humbled by how much everyone has been willing to give to make this trip possible. We thank God for each and every one of you no matter what your part in this was. We also want to thank everyone for all the uplifting prayers and support that our family has received.

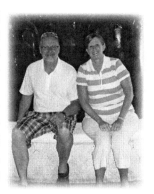

They also wanted to congratulate Western on their state championship. Jim (and Sylvia) we all know how exciting this was for you! They will be arriving home late Monday night.

Again thank you for all of your prayers and support! Mindy

Tuesday, March 20, 2007 9:07 a.m.

Over the past few days, I wondered what I would write when I finally got the opportunity to write again on my CaringBridge site. I wondered how I would thank everyone for their support, not only for the gift that helped us vacation for a few days, but for all the other support. As I grabbed my computer, I saw the cards I had received over the past few days and decided to open the cards and letters first. I was overwhelmed. The words of the cards, the hand-written notes, the wonderful "pictures" from Amira and Nico, (okay, maybe I did laugh when I saw these) and just the pure thought of others remembering me brought me to sobbing. Not tears of sorrow, but tears of gratitude, gratitude for all of you, gratitude for God's hand in placing me in such a caring community. I continue to be amazed at the variety of people who remember me, to be amazed at those who continue to keep me in their thoughts and prayers. I suppose I've said this before, but it is all of you (yes, and God) who give me strength to continue on this road.

It was wonderful to be gone for a few days. I was worried that maybe the peace and quiet of being gone would give me time to fret and worry about Thursday, the day I begin chemo, but the opposite was true. We were truly blessed with an absolutely refreshing time. The early morning walks on the beach with the water lapping at our feet, the enjoyment of a different culture, snorkeling in the reefs, and basking in the warm sun were wonderful reminders of a wonderful God, a God who made a beautiful world, one we can enjoy as well as work in. We did leave our work behind. When we left we promised each other we wouldn't do work. I don't remember the last time I left home without taking my computer, papers to correct, or books that needed to be read for school. We enjoyed each other and even (after many years of marriage) discovered things we didn't know about each other. It's been a long time since we have spent time together just focusing on each other. We also had time to talk about the future, continuing to focus on our hopes and dreams. We are very grateful for this special time we had together and continue to be humbled by the way it was provided for us.

As I think about all the ways people have given to us during the past few months, it seems symbolic of what Jesus Christ has done for us. He gave His life for us. We remember that and believe. Just as you reach for the cup and bread to celebrate Christ's great gift for us, you have also opened yourself up to us as you give in so many ways. You have been given to us by Christ to nourish and feed us. Hebrews 10:24 reads: "Let us consider how we may spur one another on toward love and good deeds." We have seen your good deeds! Peter De Vries wrote that "We are primarily put on this earth not to see through one another, but to see one another through." We are the recipients of your love.

Wednesday, March 21, 2007 8:42 a.m.

Good Morning dear friends,

I must admit last night wasn't a very restful night. Even though the doctor has assured me that the chemo treatments should not be too hard on me, I still wonder what is really going to happen. At least every hour I woke up to check the time. One of the times I lay awake longer than the others and I began to think about a book I had just finished reading—*Left To Tell*. The book was written by one of the Tutsi survivors in the Rwanda holocaust. I had left the book lying on the night stand so I turned the light on and turned to a page that I had marked while reading. The story is about a woman who, with seven other women, survived the mass killings by living in a bathroom described as a closet for 91 days. The part I'd marked tells how Immaculee survived a bout of high fever and felt that God had allowed her to survive because He had a purpose for her. Then she said something that really spoke to me. "At first I was expecting Him to show me my entire future all at once—maybe with a flash of lightning and a clap of thunder thrown in for good measure. But I came to learn that God never shows us something we aren't ready to understand. Instead, he lets us see what we need to see, when we need to see it. He'll wait until our eyes and hearts are open to Him, and then when we're ready, He will plant our feet on the path that's best for us, but it is up to us to do the walking." I guess that's what Proverbs 3:5 is all about: "Trust in the Lord with all your heart and lean not on your own understanding; in all your ways acknowledge him, and he will make your paths straight." I'm ready to walk the path on which He's planted my feet, and I know that He'll be with me every step of the way. I'm praying that those of you who read this find this truth helpful too.

Besides continuing to pray for my mom and dad who are struggling with health issues, and for my sister who gets another treatment today, I've added one of my aunts to my prayer list. At her doctor's appointment yesterday, they discovered a lump in her breast. If you've got a little room on your prayer list, I know they'd appreciate your prayers. Blessings to you today as you walk in His steps. Loving all of you.

Thursday, March 22, 2007 6:53 a.m.

I've always known that God is a God of power and mystery but yesterday He showed me His wondrous love in remarkable ways. After my restless night, I spent the morning wrestling with anxious thoughts. Questions flooded my mind. What if I get to the clinic and they find a reason to reschedule the treatments? What if I react to the drugs? How will I feel after the treatment? Will I really be able to teach next week? But I didn't have much time to fret. Before I knew it, I was greeted with encouraging conversations and e-mails, hugs, notes and chocolate, lunch with a friend, pats on the back, assurance of prayers, coffee with my parents, telephone calls, beautiful notes from the young people and their leaders of our church, more calls, visitors who kept me laughing and focusing on things other than the day ahead, and late e-mails that gave me food for thought.

As I visited with our minister tonight, I had to admit that if I could pinch myself and wake up to find out that this whole thing is a dream, I would say, "Thank God." But, when I think about it, I have to admit that through this all, I have said many, many times, "Thank You, God." Thank You God for friends, for acquaintances, for e-mails, for cards and letters, for visitors, for words of encouragement, for prayers! I've come to realize that without this trial, I would have never gotten to know some of you. Thank You God for filling up my days so that I was too busy to worry. Without this trial, I wouldn't have been able to see the many ways God's people step up to the plate and find ways to support each other. Without this trial, I would have never been reminded of the wonderful ways God shows His love for me and how He shows me who He is. It may take a while for me truly to be able to thank God for this trial, but in the meantime, He is blessing me in immeasurable ways. Isaiah 30:18 reads, "Yet the LORD longs to be gracious to you; he rises to show you compassion. For the Lord is a God of justice. Blessed are all who wait for him."

We're off to Sioux Falls. I'll begin with some blood work at 8:30 and then chemo at 9:00. The doctor is anticipating that the treatment will last approximately four hours. I should be quite comfortable sitting in a recliner in the infusion room that is run by three wonderful nurses. I'm thankful Jerry will be taking me for this first treatment. Please pray that it is successful. Thank you.

Friday, March 23, 2007 10:43 a.m.

Good Morning,

God's mystery is truly overwhelming. Each day I receive His over-flowing blessings. I suppose it is always that way but the blessings were so obvious to me yesterday. To begin with, Jerry and I had a nice quiet ride to Sioux Falls. We watched for birds and patches of green grass. Even though we weren't very successful, it helped pass the time quickly. My only anxious time was when I realized I was wearing a turtleneck and wondered if that would hinder the access to my port. We quickly stopped at Lewis Drug and all I could find was an ugly shirt for $7.00 that would match my pants, so the Dutchman in me nixed that idea. I figured if I had to, I'd wear one of those delightful gowns, but I found out that turtlenecks work too.

When we reached the cancer center, Jerry dropped me off, parked the car, and went to wait at the elevator doors. A woman walked up and said, "You are Josh's dad, aren't you." She didn't ask, she stated it. Jerry was surprised and before he could come up with her name, she said, "I'm Lorna." Lorna had been Josh's nurse fourteen years ago when Josh was in McKennan healing from his head injury. Jerry was, of course, shocked but no more shocked than I when they walked off the elevator together. As I said yesterday, God does work in mysterious ways—Lorna was like an angel to us when Josh was hospitalized. She gave superb care, advo-cated for us every step of the way, laughed with us, cried with us, and supported us in our decisions. We were hit with a flood of emotions at the sight of her. She told us of her journey with cancer which saddened our hearts; she had cervical cancer that has now spread to her chest wall, but she has had other cancers in between. I can't imagine all the anxiety and worry this wonderful lady has experienced the past five years. Even through all her trials, she was like an angel to us again yesterday. She helped us understand the procedures, sat with us through the wait, gave us good advice, and all with a huge smile on her face. We are still in shock over the many ways that God uses others to comfort us.

God promises us this, but sometimes we don't see it or believe it enough to see it. "God is not a man, that he should lie, nor a son of man, that he should change his mind. Does he speak and then not act? Does he promise and not fulfill?" (Numbers 23:19). Every day I can see God's promises if I but look around. I can also be a part of God's promises as I (as many of you have done) reach out to others. I'm going to be looking to see how I can reach out as many of you have done for me.

The treatment went even better than I could have expected. I first had labs drawn and there is always some anxiety there, because if something shows up that the doctors don't like, they can cancel your treatment. I also had a sore on my chin that I was afraid she might see as dangerous for bleeding, but that wasn't a problem and my blood came back with a go sign so it was off to the transfusion room. My port was a great blessing. No poking, no searching for veins. The first part of the treatment was issuing premeds, meds that we hoped would ward off side effects. Next they gave me Avastin. While this drug was dripping into my veins, would you believe I had a lot of company? Marcia came with some beautiful tulips (which I am now enjoying while I sit here), my Uncle Tom and Aunt Laura stopped over, and then mom and Norm (my brother) stopped in. I didn't even notice the medical things that were happening.

Then came the next premeds before Paxil. Wow! I don't remember a whole lot after that. The premed made me so sleepy I could hardly put my syllables together as I talked. I felt foolish asking for help to the bathroom, but I wasn't sure I could put one foot in front of the other. That was it for me. I sat back in that chair, and I don't remember much of anything until I woke up this morning. I'm still not sure how I got into the car and then into the house when we got home. I'm feeling fine this morning, just a little sluggish and slow. I hope to go for a walk pretty soon. Maybe by drinking full glasses of water and doing some exercise, I can move the drug through my body.

Thanks for all the prayers. I could feel myself, each step of the way, being carried on the wings of eagles. What a blessing.

Saturday, March 24, 2007 8:54 a.m.

Good Morning,

Yesterday was a beautiful day, full of sunshine and warm air. After I finally awoke from my deep sleep, I went outside to rake the leaves off my flower beds. It felt good to do some physical work and I was thrilled to see the new green shoots popping out of the ground. I thought of the verse that Laura quoted: "See! The winter is past; the rains are over and gone. Flowers appear on the earth; the season of singing has come"(Song of Songs 2:11-12). As I cleaned around those new sprouts, I could only imagine what they will grow to be in a few short weeks. I can just see the brightly colored tulips mixed with the light pastels. I was struck by two thoughts as my hands dug around the base of the new plants, pulling away the rotting debris: I hoped that as the new plants are growing, so are the healthy cells in my lung. I thought of the medicine loosening up the bad cells and getting rid of them. I appreciated Kim's prayer for the chemo to begin working. It reminded me of a conversation Megan and I had while I was walking. I began to cough and we wondered if maybe the medicine was starting to work on the nodule, a little early I would guess, but who knows.

It also made me think of my life here on earth. I am like a plant. I have been given my life to live in obedience to God. Sometimes my life becomes stale and doesn't produce much, but at other times I flourish and produce the kinds of things God wants me to. The springtime is a good reminder for me to check my growth. Do others see new shoots growing out of me? Do people recognize my vibrant colors? I hope my life represents the New Life that God has planted inside of me. An aside: As a beautiful reminder of what little green shoots can become, my friend Pat sent me a beautiful bouquet of flowers to remind me of what my garden will become and what I need to aim for in my life.

I'm really tired today. I didn't sleep well until I finally resigned myself to needing a sleeping pill for which the doctor had written a prescription. After that I did sleep but am feeling exhausted. I hope more energy will return throughout the day. Thank you for your prayers and encouragements. They've come in many "packages," and we've appreciated every one of them.

Sunday, March 25, 2007 12:25 p.m.

As I lay thinking in bed this morning, I wondered what the day would be like. Yesterday was one of those days where the ride just seemed to dip deeper and deeper as the day went. I was achy when I got up, my throat and neck hurt, and I felt exhausted. It didn't help my emotions that I had read the night before that some patients were being pulled off Avastin, the drug I had injected into me on Thursday. There seems to be some concern about the drug causing perforations in the gastrointestinal tract. I'll be talking to my doctor about this tomorrow. The doctor did tell us that the pre-drugs do contain some uppers and some downers which help for a host of other things but don't always keep the emotions in check. That's what it was like for me. I could (and did) cry about any-thing. Poor Jerry didn't know what to do with me until he decided it was time to give me something to counter the weepiness. It at least helped me fall asleep. I knew even if I was tired this morning, I wanted to go to church, plus I had no choice: I was on the schedule to play. I wanted to go to worship God, the giver of my life and I did, but oh, the blessings He sent my way far outweighed what I gave to Him. How can one not find comfort while singing "What A Friend We Have in Jesus." "Are we weak and heavy laden, cumbered with a load of care? Precious Savior, still our refuge! Take it to the Lord in prayer. In His arms He'll take and shield you; you will find a solace there." When I'm struggling to feel His arms around me, all I need to do is take it to my Lord in prayer. What a blessing it is to be in His presence. Enjoy your day, reflecting on and worshiping a Great, Big, Mighty God!

Monday, March 26, 2007 9:24 a.m.

> Fill my cup Lord, Fill it up, Lord
> Oh, fill my cup, fill my cup, let it overflow.
> Oh, fill my cup, fill my cup, let it overflow.
> Oh, fill my cup, fill my cup,
> let it overflow, let it overflow with love.

Those were the words I used to teach to every student in my elemen-tary classroom. Before we sang this song, we would often talk about how our cups could overflow. This conversation often took place before our Bible lesson, so it was quite natural for the students to answer that study-ing God's Word was one way for them to fill their cups. As we considered these words, we often talked about how the "cup filling" was spiritual.

This weekend, I believe, I found another meaning. I discovered that in order to be able to overflow with a spiritual love, one must have physi-cal strength. Another lesson in this life. This weekend I struggled physi-cally—not with nausea or achy bones, but with a feeling of emptiness, a feeling of anxiety. And just as God promises, He was there beside me. Jerry skipped a banquet so he could be with me, my children's conversa-tions lifted me, the flowers on my mantle were a brightener, the church service helped me take a better look at who God is, and playing ball with my grandsons on Sunday also helped to fill my cup. I often tell my col-lege students that they need to make sure that their students' physical and emotional "cups" are full in order for them to have a full spiritual cup.

After my experience this weekend, I'm even more convinced. Our minister gave the example of a sponge; when it sits in a pan of water, it sucks up all the water. I'm like that too: I need to soak myself in God's Word and in all the other opportunities He provides in order to overflow with love. Today I am asking God to fill my cup, to give me the strength and emotional stability so that I can let my cup overflow for Him. Thanks for the many ways you have filled my cup and the cups of others around you.

Tuesday, March 27, 2007 8:09 a.m.

Good Morning,

As I walked out my front door and headed for my dirt road along which I often walk, I realized that it didn't take a rocket scientist to notice the change that has happened over the past few months. The snow piles are gone, the strong cold north wind has changed, there's water running through the drainage pipes, and the birds are singing joyful songs. I, being a fair-weather person, loved the change. It was wonderful to feel the crunch of the gravel under my feet. And even though I didn't move with the stride of a runner, it felt good to breathe in the warm air and feel my muscles stretch with each step. As I turned the corner to head down the lonely stretch of road, I was struck by the change in my life too. In the last couple of months I've had a breast removed, a port inserted, my schedule changed, my dreams put on hold, and my certainty shaken. The two seemed in sharp contrast with each other. As I gently kicked the stones that stood in my way, I contemplated the joy of the one change and the apprehension of the other. Would I want the first picture to have stayed the same: cold wintry weather with snow all over? Most definitely not! What about the second scene? Would I like my life to rewind to the early part of January and start over with a new scenario? Part of me says, "Yes," but in my heart, I know that the road I'm on is the road I have to travel. I don't know why and maybe I never will, but I know that it is the one that is mine. But the beauty of this road is that it isn't lonely, it is full of joy and blessings. When I look back toward the beginning of the road, I can't begin to count all the blessings that have come my way. I see God walking right beside me. I see friends and family supporting me. I see doctors, nurses, and technicians who have helped cushion every curve that came my way. And I'm just started. I don't know what the future holds. I don't know what lessons I will learn or maybe what lessons you will learn, or who will see God's glory through all of this, but I do know who holds the future and I'm going to trust in Him.

Matthew 6:25-27 says this:

Therefore I tell you, do not worry about your life, what you will eat or drink; or about your body, what you will wear. Is not life more important than food, and the body more important than clothes? Look at the birds of the air; they do not sow or reap or store away in barns, and yet your heavenly Father feeds them. Are you not much more valuable than they? Who of you by worrying can add a single hour to his life?

I hope you are able to enjoy the beauty not only of the outdoors but of the life that God has given to you. If you have worries, take them to the Lord, the One who holds your future, and rely on Him to give you what you need today.

I'm hoping to get some school work done today. I am scheduled for three meetings tonight. It feels good to be juggling schedules once again. I've called the doctor about the drug Avastin that was in the news and she, at this point, is not worried and says I will continue on it. I have to call her about a cough I've developed, but I don't want anything to stand in the way of my treatment on Thursday. Blessings to all of you,

Wednesday, March 28, 2007 8:23 a.m.

I'm already behind and it is only 8:20. I'll write a little later today. I hope you are having a good day.

Wednesday, March 28, 2007 10:46 a.m.

It was one of those days. Morning came too quickly. I didn't want to get out of bed. My head hurt and my body ached. But I crawled out and found that the shower did some good in waking up my mind and body. But it continued—I left my cell phone at home, forgot my lunch, and missed the corner on the bypass. And then I walked up the steps in my office building and I saw the print of a beautiful rising sun and written on it was the very last part of Psalm 30:5: ". . . but rejoicing comes in the morning." You bet. I'm rejoicing that there is a morning, a day to proclaim God's faithfulness. A day that can be turned into dancing and cause my heart to sing and not be silent. "O Lord my God, I will give you thanks forever" (vs. 12). I hope that even on this rainy day, you can find reason to sing and dance.

Thursday, March 29, 2007 6:55 a.m.

You know how a mind can wander? You begin with something in your presence and before you know it you've leaped across miles of "acreage." That's how it was for me as I sat in my office chair yesterday. I read something about roots and that got me to thinking about trees and that lead to water, then the lake, and then my brother and his father-in-law's experience on the beach of their once-owned cabin on Silver Lake.

You see, there was this beautiful tree that stood between the cabin and the lake. It provided much appreciated shade and it added to the beautiful landscape. Shortly after a storm ripped through the area, Norm, my brother, and his father-in-law, Louie Kuiper, went up to the cabin to check for any damages that might have occurred. Much to their happiness, the cabin had survived the storm in good shape, but as they rounded the building, to their dismay, they found that the beautiful ash tree had been flattened. Not knowing what else to do and realizing that it couldn't stay on the beach, they decided to cut the tree into firewood. They revved up the saws and each began cutting the short top branches of the tree. They progressed down the trunk of the tree, each working on a side. They were getting quite a nice bundle of wood for firewood. Each was thoughtfully doing his job, when all of a sudden, the tree jumped and stood in its rightful place, just as straight but a little shorter than the day before. What had happened is that the roots had just been stretched. When the top of the tree was made lighter by cutting off the branches, the strong roots took control and pulled that tree right up again. We've often laughed about that story. We would have loved to have seen Mr. Kuiper and Norm in their flight to get out of the way of that "jumping" tree. It must have been a pretty funny sight.

It seems to me that this is a great representation of what happens in our lives. We often get bogged down by heavy weights. Some days I can look at life with doubt, negative thoughts, dissatisfaction, fear, and worry. I get bogged down. When I let those negative thoughts go, my load lightens, and I too can stand tall and do the work that God has called me to do. I love what Jeremiah says to us in chapter 17:7-8: "But blessed is the man who trusts in the LORD, whose confidence is in him. He will be like a tree planted by the water that sends out its roots by the stream. It does not fear when heat comes; its leaves are always green. It has no worries in the year of drought and never fails to bear fruit." It takes a lot of work to grow those roots deep, but God blesses the effort with a fruitful tree.

I'm on my way for another round of chemo. I'm praying that this treatment goes as well as the first. Thanks again for all the wonderful ways you continue to show your fruitfulness to us. Tonight I came home late from school to find a fridge full of food. Ladies from the church had dropped off the leftover Lenten luncheon food. Jerry is once again well-fed. I'm thankful for friends who will drive me to Sioux Falls—today it is my friend Lorna. I'm thankful for my students who showed up to class wearing pink ribbons to show their support for me and I'm thankful for my colleagues who continue to support me. I'm also thankful for all those Western Christian Chamber Singers who blessed me with hugs, even after I missed their program. So many of you continue to raise my spirits and keep me hopeful. Thank You.

Friday, March 30, 2007 7:28 a.m.

Yesterday I had my second of the three treatments in the first series of chemo. Right now Dr. Krie anticipates three of these series and then she'll do a PET scan to see what is happening with the spot on my lung. From there she will decide what to do next. It could be more of the same; it all depends on what the test shows. I really appreciate Dr. Krie. She is honest and forthright. She tells me like it is. As usual, today she told me some things I didn't want to hear, but she was also more positive about the possibility of complete healing. The good news that Dr. Krie shared today is that the drug Avastin has improved survival rates by 50%. She was very encouraged by the way my body reacted to the treatments. She was impressed with my counts. She did cut back on one of the premeds that really sedated me last week and I actually slept only through the chemo treatment. Before I fell asleep, we had quite a little party going. Three of us sat in a row, receiving our chemo—my Sioux Falls friend Lorna, my twin sister Marcia, and me—with Lorna's husband Dave, Jerry's sister Shar and another friend of mine, Lorna, sitting across from us entertaining us with great conversation. I hope we didn't take over the place too much. I tried to stay in the conversation as long as I could but I didn't last long. Before I knew it they were waking me up, telling me that my chemo was finished. I was able to stay awake for the ride home and had a great evening getting some work finished.

Back to Dr. Krie. As much as I love her, I know that Dr. Krie isn't going to heal me; doctors don't do that; only God can do that. We have a wonderful example of this in II Kings 5. It's the story of the little slave girl who cared about her master Naaman enough to suggest a healer for his leprosy. "If only my master would see the prophet who is in Samaria! He would cure him of his leprosy," the little girl told Naaman's wife. Amazingly Naaman listened to the little girl, traveled to another country to see a prophet he had never heard of, and was cured. In my case God can use doctors to help heal my body. I believe God sent Dr. Krie to Sioux Falls just in time for her to be my physician, to try a new treatment that is showing great results. The God of all hope has led me to a doctor who has given me hope for healing in my journey with cancer.

"But now, Lord, what do I look for? My hope is in you" (Psalm 39:7). I thank God the ultimate healer, and I also thank Him for sending many great people who are helping to heal me.

Saturday, March 31, 2007 8:02 a.m.

Good Day,

Today's journal is probably the hardest journal I've written up to this point. Today is the first of two fundraisers that family and friends are putting on for us. Some might ask, why so close together. Well, unbeknownst to us, our friends and our children both planned something without the other knowing. When they came to us with the plans already in place, we didn't know what to say or how to choose one. So, two fund raisers in three days. It's not that I'm not thankful; I am very thankful for the many people who are willing to give up their time and have put their effort into the fund raisers. I'm very thankful for those who have shown an interest in supporting them, so then I have to ask myself, why am I bothered? Why am I bothered? Why does it make me emotional? I'm emotional, I think, because of the pure gratitude I feel, gratitude for the emotional and financial help. It is a humbling experience to feel the care and love of this many people. It is almost overwhelming. So is that the reason for my nervousness? Is it a matter of pride—what if no one comes? Or is it a matter of never being very good at receiving? Oh, I've received plenty in my life, but never like now. My mother has reminded me throughout my life that this was one area I could work on—receiving graciously. (She told me kindly.) One area she would remind me that I needed to work on was accepting compliments graciously. You see, I had a habit of justifying compliments that I would receive. If the compliment concerned a piece of clothing I was wearing, I would say that my mom had made it for me or that I had gotten a really good deal. If people complimented me on work that I had accomplished, I had a difficult time simply saying, "Thanks." So maybe that has laid the foundation for why it is difficult for me to know how to handle all this giving that is coming to me.

Paul tells us in Acts 20:35: "In everything I did, I showed you that by this kind of hard work we must help the weak, remembering the words the Lord Jesus himself said: 'It is more blessed to give than to receive.'" We all know this is true, but living in a culture in which we pride ourselves in thinking we are people who have it all together, who pride ourselves in our independence, who have been taught to be self-sufficient, it isn't easy merely to accept. Maybe receiving makes me feel as if I'm desolate or maybe it's a big reminder of what I'm going through or what is ahead. I still don't have this whole thing figured out, but I do know one thing, I am grateful! I'm very thankful for those who have spent much time putting together and working at the pancake supper and auction. I'm thankful for those who donated items and for those who will purchase them. I'm thankful for the Pizza Ranch managers for giving part of the proceeds of Monday night to us, for those who will serve at it, and for those who will eat pizza at the Pizza Ranch. I know I've used this song before, but it seems to applicable again:

> "The Servant Song"
> Brother, sister, let me serve you,
> Let me be as Christ to you;
> Pray that I may have the grace to let you be my servant too.

The third verse seems to sum up much of what I've felt from you over the past months.

> I will weep when you are weeping;
> When you laugh, I'll laugh with you.
> I will share your joy and sorrow
> Till we see this journey through.

Thanks for all your past and continuing support. I love you all!

Saturday, March 31, 2007 1:24 p.m.

Many people have asked today about the benefits. This evening there will be a pancake supper and auction at the Sanborn Christian School in Sanborn beginning at 5 p.m. On Monday night, April 2, there will be a benefit at the Pizza Ranch in Sheldon from 5-7:30. Thanks for all your love.

Monday, April 2, 2007 8:33 a.m.

After busy days Saturday and Sunday, I'm back to my website. Yesterday I had the privilege of playing the morning service with Catherine Schreur and her sister Cheyenne Heath. After church we went to my parents' home for dinner; only a few family members were missing so their house was full and noisy, a wonderful way to spend Palm Sunday.

Some of you may be wondering how I survived last Saturday. It was a wonderful night! Between some spurts of emotionalism, I held it together pretty well. It was shocking to see all the people who came out, but it was also a joy to be able to talk to many friends and hear their encouraging words and especially to hear about all the prayers that were being said on my behalf. What a blessing! People were truly gracious.

Many of our friends worked hard to make the fund raisers happen. They set up for the supper; they organized gifts; they managed the meal, and they cleaned up. What a lot of work for all of them. There were others, but it was Jerry's snowmobile club that did the bulk of the work. We want to thank them from the bottom of our hearts. We also want to thank all those who came to the supper. Colleagues, old friends, new friends, students whom I had taught in the past, neighbors, church friends, town people, acquaintances, and more. We were shocked at the turnout.

And then the auction. Many people donated beautiful and useful items. At one time I was so overwhelmed that I wondered who would buy all the items. But by the end of the night, everything had disappeared into the wonderful hands of supporters. One of the best surprises of the night was the appearance of the Chamber Singers of Western Christian. I was invited to their fund raiser last week, but because of a prior commitment, I missed most of the performance. Jerry, being the planner and "surpriser" that he is, asked the kids if they would come and sing a few songs before the auction began. What an emotional roller coaster that was. You find out you can cry, laugh, and enjoy all at one time. I would like to thank all those young people who took time out of their Saturday night activities to bless me. Their songs were beautifully sung, but even more importantly carried a message that spoke to me.

I have to get to teaching so I need to go—I'll write more later, but I wanted to share this verse when thinking about the graciousness of God's people: "Be joyful always; pray continually; give thanks in all circumstances, for this is God's will for you in Christ Jesus." I experienced much joy this weekend; I prayed continually that God would walk beside me through this beautiful act of kindness; and He certainly did. I continue to give thanks in all my circumstances. Have a good day!

Tuesday, April 3, 2007 9:11 a.m.

Last night was another overwhelming night. We were again completely amazed at the support that we experienced at the Pizza Ranch fund raiser. Thank you to all who came and to those who helped by cleaning and bussing tables. What a workout you had! We appreciate all the time you gave. Thanks also to Nate Breen and the Sheldon Pizza Ranch for helping to make this possible. It was wonderful to be able to talk to many students, friends and family members. It was great fun reminiscing with you. By the end of the evening I was exhausted, but it was a good kind of exhaustion. Many of you assured me that you continue to pray—what a blessing! Your prayers are something we have coveted from the beginning of this journey, and we continue to appreciate the time you spend in prayer on our behalf.

I read an article recently titled "What Are Friends For." It talked about the healing process that friends (and family) bring and how important it is to surround yourself with friends who are willing to be there for you. The article talked about not needing rationalization or explanation. Friends are just there! They laugh with you, cry with you, encourage you, are quiet with you, are noisy with you, hold you, pray for you, and love you. (I'm sure there are more descriptives.) And what is incredible is that God sends each of you our way with new and different ways to encourage. Good friends are invaluable. But there is one friend who does it all.

Proverbs 18:24 says: ". . . there is a friend that sticks closer than a brother." I'm thankful for all of you, and I'm also thankful for my Heavenly "friend" who watches over me day and night.

Thanks for your support. As I said Saturday night, we thank God for the support we have been given, and we are praying that we will use the gifts given to us with wisdom and discernment.

Even on this gloomy day, enjoy the day. Bring some sunshine into someone's life.

Thursday, April 5, 2007 7:37 a.m.

As you may have noticed, I was absent from the CaringBridge site for a day. Wow! Teaching has made a difference in my life. I'm thankful to be back in the classroom. People constantly ask me how it's going, and I always reply, "Great, but you might want to ask my students. They may see it differently." I'm enjoying every minute of it. Yesterday my daughter Megan met with some students interested in pursuing the child-life profession. I thought that those of you at De Vos might want to know that she did a fantastic job. The college students were very eager to hear what she had to say.

The weather here in N'West Iowa has been miserable the past few days. It seems as if we are going backward in seasons rather than forward. The past few days have been full of blasting winds. Amira and I ran up a hill yesterday and I held onto her firmly because I was afraid she would be blown off the path. As I was lying in bed, listening to those strong blasts, I wondered how much the "wind" in my life has affected me. How much has the cultural wind of the day swayed me? How much has the "materialistic" wind of today influenced me? How much has the "desire to succeed" wind driven me? Even now, how much does the "wind of doubt" pattern the way I think? The wind is strong and powerful. It has a lot of influence. It makes a person tired when working in it. It has the power to destroy. It decides what kind of clothes I'm going to wear. It decides if I'm going to walk outdoors. It is very influential. So it is with winds in our lives. We can be controlled by winds that influence in sinful ways. Or we can be influenced by the Wind of the Spirit. He works in ways we can't predict or understand.

Josh and Mike very graciously covered my gardens with coverings on that first cold night. We decided that even tulips might have a difficult time with that cold wind. They anchored each of the corners to be sure the wind didn't whip the covering off. We too must be covered by God's Word. This doesn't happen by our doings but by the work of the Spirit that He sends. In order for us to hear God's voice and feel the Spirit working, we must be covered with the righteousness of God which comes to us through the anchors of life. Just as those rocks held the cover in place, so God's Word anchors us into knowing Him and His ways.

It's calm today (at least so far). I hope we have all withstood that raging wind and can now enjoy the beauty of the calm in God's physical and spiritual world.

Megan, Mindy, and I are leaving in a few minutes for Sioux Falls for my last treatment in this first set. Next week I have a free week before I begin my next series. I'm praying that God will continue to bless these treatments both as I receive them today and as they work in my body. I'm trusting Him to help the medicine work. Have a calm day.

Thursday, April 5, 2007 11:04 p.m.

Whoa, what a day! I've enjoyed everyone who has willingly taken me to my chemo appointments thus far, but it was an extra blessing having my daughters with me at my appointment today. They caused quite a stir! At one point I was worried about them getting kicked out of the infusion room, for, shall I say, expressing their abundance of joy. They had the nurses and other patients in a stitch. I even saw one nurse whom I haven't seen smile much, giggle quietly in her work area. My doctor even got in on some of the action after she proclaimed what beautiful daughters I have. I know she could see their inner beauty as well as their outer beauty. That makes a mother proud! I also had another blessing today. Roger and Karen Koole read on my CaringBridge site that I was having another treatment today so they surprised me with a visit during my treatment. What beautiful and encouraging people these new friends are. We met the Koole's through Mr. Van Soelen, our kids' high school principal and our friend. Roger is just finishing his cancer treatments. Our new friendship with the Koole's is one of the many examples of the wonderful connections we've made through our journey.

I know I've mentioned this before, but think with me for a moment. I would love to go back to January 12 and change the news we got from the doctor. However, I know in my heart that as difficult as this is, I wouldn't want to give up the many blessings I've experienced the past two months. I received a short devotional in the mail today from a dear friend Carolyn Bootsma. It was titled *Only One You* by John Fischer. I was struck by a few lines toward the end of the writing. After the author reminded his readers of our uniqueness and yet our responsibility to live for the Body of Christ, he wrote:

> And then think about the things you have gone through so far in your life—especially the difficult or challenging things where God has met you with his presence and power. That information is not just for you, it's for you to empathize with and encourage others who have encountered similar struggles. God doesn't mess around. There are no accidents with our lives. Whatever we have received and experienced has shaped who we are, and because of that, we are qualified servants.

Thank you for empathizing with me and for the ways you've acted on the qualifications God has given you. Thank you for letting me share with all of you. "The body is a unit, though it is made up of many parts; and though all its parts are many, they form one body. So it is with Christ . . . . Now you are the body of Christ, and each of you is a part of it" (I Corinthians 12:12, 27). Blessings to you as you serve the Body.

Saturday, April 7, 2007 9:37 a.m.

"HELP, Megan, come here!" That's how my day began yesterday. I woke up feeling amazingly good, even after a restless night. Dr. Krie was again very happy with my response to treatments. My counts continue to look good although my white count had dropped some, so to ensure that it stayed up until I came back, she ordered a shot that produces mega white cells. She said it might make me achy in my joints, which would require another medication, but so far I feel fine.

Anyway, back to the hair episode. I was getting ready for school.

Megan had stayed overnight because of our late return from Sioux Falls. I had just finished combing my hair when I looked down and saw that my shirt was covered with hair. I tugged—not very hard—and handfuls came falling out. I didn't know whether to cry or laugh. I knew I couldn't stand there all day and pull on my hair, so with assurance from Megan that I looked alright, we left for Sioux Center. All morning I tried to keep my fingers out of my hair, but every once in a while I would catch myself with my fingers wrapped around some hair, and sure enough, out would come some more. I had been warned that this would eventually happen but I guess nothing can prepare you for it. I've never really enjoyed doing my hair so it wasn't that. I'm usually envious of Jerry who gets up later than I but often leaves the house before me because all he has to do is run his fingers through his hair.

I think it is the feeling of loss and a realization that there is a sickness in my body. Up until this time, I really haven't felt the effects of cancer. I've felt the effects of surgery and medicine that are needed to control the disease, but nothing from the cancer. The hair loss is also a result of drugs rather than cancer, but it is a visible sign that something unnatural is going on in my body. I left school as soon as I was finished teaching, not knowing what I might look like later that day. Anyway, just as I was starting to feel sorry for myself, a beautiful plant arrived from my sister-in-law with note to perk me up. Then a beautiful fresh flower arrangement arrived from my friend Pat with a note telling me that I am beautiful with or without hair. Amazing how self pity can turn around. I was grateful for these two outward displays of love that helped me put perspective back into the picture. I may be losing my hair, but that doesn't change who I am. I can no longer trust my body to produce hair, but I can trust God to take care of me. Flowers are such a sign of life and the two gifts reminded me that I still have life, life to give to God and to others. Right now I am receiving much from others, but I hope that soon I can return these acts of kindness. I am trusting God to bring me to that day. Last night I was also reminded of all the prayers that are going up to God for me.

I was telling my friend Alvina about the amazing way my body is reacting to the drugs and she said, "It's all those prayers that are being said for you." I knew people were praying but it was good to be reminded of that. Thanks for all your prayers. Bernard M. Baruch once said, "The art of living lies less in eliminating your troubles than in growing with them." I hope this "trouble" helps me grow in the art of living. Blessings to all of you during this very special season of the year when we ache, knowing the pain that Christ suffered for us but also knowing the joy we experience through His resurrection.

Monday, April 9, 2007 5:39 a.m.

Good Morning,

Easter weekend is one of my favorite times of the year. For me it began with a meaningful Good Friday service in the chapel at Dordt and concluded with my De Wit cousins acting as living sacrifices. Let me explain. Our chapel service at Dordt included "reading" the story of Christ's death from each of the four gospels. One gospel was read from scripture, one was done from memory, one as a Reader's Theater, and one was enacted by mime. It was a powerful way of being reminded of God's love and Christ's sacrifice for us. On Friday evening we attended the Tenebrae service at our church. At the end of the service, the extinguished candles reminded me of the sin of the world and then the re-entry of the Christ candle emphasized the hope of His promised resurrection. Even though Good Friday services often leave me with a heavy feeling, they also lead to the great joy of Easter morning. We woke to an unseasonably cold morning on Sunday, but the beautiful bright sunshine was a great reminder of the Light of the World who rose centuries ago to bring us eternal life. In church we were reminded that Christ's victory, His crown of thorns changed to a crown of glory, was for us and through it all, we too shall receive a crown of glory (Philippians 2:9-11).

After church we enjoyed a delicious meal at Kim and Ed's where we once again felt the love and support of family. And then in the evening, Mar and John and Larry and Aud (my cousins), stopped over and showered us with a wonderful basket of goodies. It symbolized to us the living sacrifice that God calls each of us to. It reminded me of Paul's command in Ephesians 5:1-2: "Be imitators of God, therefore, as dearly loved children and live a life of love, just as Christ loved us and gave himself up for us as a fragrant offering and sacrifice to God."

It was a timely weekend for me. As far as my health, the past weekend was probably the most difficult since surgery. It began on Friday with my hair falling out (which, by the way, has just thinned so far and not completely fallen out), continued with extreme fatigue on Saturday, and then on Sunday the body ache hit me. It was a pulsating pain that radiated through my body every time I moved. Dr. Krie had warned me that the shot to increase my white cell count could do this and wow did it. It began Sunday morning with an ache in my back and increasingly got worse until I finally called the doctor in the evening. The on-call doctor was very helpful and gave me great advice that helped relieve the pain somewhat. He also said that the pain was evidence that the shot was doing what they had hoped it would so that made the pain more bearable.

As I said, the weekend was timely. Throughout the weekend, even though I didn't feel well, I was constantly reminded of God's love for me. I heard of His love through the services we attended and once again witnessed His love through others, not only through acts of kindness but over and over again hearing from others that they were praying for me. How amazing! How thankful I am for my Father's deep love for me, a love beyond all measure; a love that gave His only Son to make a wretch his treasure—words from "How Deep the Father's Love for Us."

My prayer is that I can live out Christ's love for me as I travel through another week. Have a wonderful week.

Tuesday, April 10, 2007 9:14 a.m.

Our youngest grandson Miles is a very special little guy (just like our other grandchildren). I know he loves us but sometimes he has a difficult time showing it. He is quite attached to his mom and dad so he likes to spend most of his time with them. The other night Mindy and Sou were invited to a program that didn't include children so that meant Miles had to be separated from his parents. Mindy and Sou dropped the boys off at Sou's brother and sister-in-law, Shawn and Stephanie. They knew there could be problems but hoped for the best. As soon as they left the house, Miles began to cry. Bailey, who is four, immediately took to comforting Miles. He went to sit on the couch and coaxed Miles to come to him. Miles climbed up on the couch, rested his head on Bailey's chest, and soon went to sleep. Bailey held him for awhile and then he carefully slipped out from under Miles. He told Steph that he was going to go and play with the other kids, but if Miles should wake up, she should come and get him right away and he would take care of his baby brother. And so he did. As soon as Miles woke up, he was right there beside him again, assuring his baby brother that things were okay. Miles was happy to have the assurance of a familiar face and spent the rest of the evening quite happy under the care of Bailey and, of course, his aunt.

Sometimes I feel that way. Like Miles, I also feel afraid, but I don't have to. Just as Bailey stood ready to comfort Miles, I always have my heavenly Father right beside me ready to comfort me. He is always there. Sometimes I feel His presence more than others, not because He isn't there, but because I don't seek Him out. All I need to do is crawl into His arms and receive His comfort. There are many verses in the Bible that talk about this but Isaiah 40:11 is one of my favorites: "He tends his flock like a shepherd: He gathers the lambs in his arms and carries them close to his heart." Deuteronomy 33:27 also assures us: "The eternal God is your refuge, and underneath are the everlasting arms."

Just as Miles needed Bailey, I need God. He is supplying what I need. Yesterday was probably the most difficult day yet on this journey. I taught my first class but soon realized I wouldn't be able to teach the second one. Everything ached; the pain throbbed through my body. My head pounded and my stomach lurched. I felt fatigued. But again, God sent others to pick me up. Pam helped me pack up my things and Kim took over my class. Josh made a delivery for me and, of course, called everyone to tell them I wasn't feeling well so they could pray. My friend Amy sent flowers which joined other bouquets that picked up my spirits. Jerry doted on me, making sure I had everything I needed. I spent most of the day sleeping and even slept last night. Sleep seems to be wonderful medicine. Today the pain is mostly gone; my stomach has settled down, and I think I'm getting my energy back. I'm relying on my Father's arms to hold me until I'm ready to get going again. Thanks for your continued words of encouragement and your prayers.

Wednesday, April 11, 2007 1:25 a.m.

What weather, huh. If you know me well, you probably figured I would mention this unlikely awful spring weather. Snow in April! I know, Iowa weather is unpredictable but this is ridiculous. Every time I looked out the window yesterday, I figured I'd see the snow change to rain, but it didn't happen; the snow just kept coming. I'm looking for flowers and all I'm seeing is snow! I sometimes feel as if in my life too, not only with the cancer I've been diagnosed with, but with other things that I'd like changed too. But some things can't be changed. Just as we can't change the weather out there, we can't always change things in our life. That's where contentment comes in. Oh, it's hard! Maybe not for you but it is for me. It is easy for me to jump ahead and want things. It's not for the needs that I am desiring, but the wants that I want. The last few days, when I was fatigued and in pain, it was really difficult to feel content. Contentment is the ability to be satisfied. I wasn't satisfied with how I was feeling; I wasn't content with what I was doing, which was mostly sleeping.

But then I read the NIV commentary on Philippians 4:10-12. Paul talks about being content in all circumstances, whether in want or plenty. The commentary said that Paul focused on God's point of view and not his own. "He focused on what he was supposed to do, not what he felt he should have." Wow! What a difference! It made me think about my situation. How much am I focusing on what God wants me to do? And how do I discern what that is? I've had to give up many activities the past few months, things I loved to do. It has left me discontented. After reading Paul's words, I've had to re-think things. I'm feeling bad because I'm not doing all the things I love to do, but maybe God wants me to concentrate on other things right now, like praising Him even through this trial. Contentment. I'm going to work on it, even when I don't feel well and the weather is rotten. " . . . for I have learned to be content whatever the circumstances. I know what it is to be in need, and I know what it is to have plenty. I have learned the secret of being content in any and every situation, whether well fed or hungry, whether living in plenty or in want. I can do everything through him who gives me strength" (Philippians 4:11b-13). I'm thankful that I've begun to feel better. About six o'clock last night my energy started to return and my body began to be rid of the pain. I'm thankful I had a day where I could just rest—the snow made me satisfied to stay indoors and enjoy the flowers that decorate my living room. I am eager to go back to school today and teach. I hope your day is full of contentment.

Thursday, April 12, 2007 2:00 a.m.

What a bummer of a day. How often have you said that the past few days while you waited for the snow to stop and the sunshine and warm temperatures to reappear? I have to admit I've said that phrase a few times myself. Sometimes it was related to how I was feeling and sometimes it was due to my feelings for the un-spring-like weather. It's probably how my Aunt Laura would describe the day she found out that the lump in her breast was cancer. I know my sister Marcia described the day she lost her hair as a bummer. My Uncle John (we called him Dutch) De Wit's family may have called yesterday a bummer. It was the day their husband, father, grandfather, and great-grandfather breathed his last breath and passed from this life to his eternal home. He left this earth a little before 7:00 a.m. With no one present, with no fanfare. It was quiet in his room. But what happened as he slipped from here to there? What excitement did he experience? We don't know. The Bible gives us few clues about heaven but isn't very descriptive of the life hereafter. To tell you the truth, I've sort of avoided thinking of heaven the past few months. Just before January I had begun to read *Heaven* by Randy Alcorn but since the diagnosis, I've put the book on hold. I'm not ready for it yet. That doesn't mean that I don't look forward to heaven, but right now I'm still loving my work here on earth. I hope that doesn't sound selfish but grateful for a wonderful life that God allowed for me to have, a life I would love to continue for a while yet.

I would imagine that Uncle Dutch isn't describing his life right now as a bummer. His family has already begun to miss him. They will miss his presence, his jokes, the love they felt from him, his conversations, etc., and they will continue to miss him. That's the bummer part. The wonderful thing is all the memories which they hold on to. I have memories too. Some of my favorite memories were swinging on the rope in the big barn and playing Monopoly in the little house. And the glorious part is that Uncle Dutch is in a beautiful place, a place which we cannot describe because we don't know what its glory is like. But we do know at least two things for sure: Heaven will be bright and vibrant, free from sin, suffering, and death and brimming with Christ's presence, and with the richness as God intended for it. It is a great contrast to the quiet little hospital room he just left. And we know that the promise of heaven is ours if we confess God to be our Lord and Savior and live a life as His servant, in gratitude for what He has done for us. Uncle Dutch left a quiet room; he left pain and suffering; he left a sinful world and entered into a world we can only imagine.

MercyMe sings a song that takes away that bummer feeling and gives us the joy that God intended for us when we think of our loved ones going to heaven. I heard this song first at my Uncle Floyd's funeral and later at one of my best friends, Pam Kreykes's funeral. I hope my uncle's family gets an opportunity to read these words as they face the next few days of saying goodbye.

> I can only imagine what it will be like, when I walk by Your side.
> I can only imagine, what my eyes will see, when Your face is before me!
> I can only imagine. I can only imagine.
>
> Surrounded by Your Glory, what will my heart feel?
> Will I dance for you, Jesus? Or in awe of You, be still?
> Will I stand in Your presence, or to my knees will I fall?
> Will I sing 'Hallelujah!'? Will I be able to speak at all?
> I can only imagine! I can only imagine!
>
> I can only imagine, when that day comes,
> when I find myself standing in the Son!
> I can only imagine, when all I will do, is forever, forever worship You!
> I can only imagine! I can only imagine!

Surrounded by Your glory, what will my heart feel?
I can only imagine, when all I do is forever, forever worship You!
I can only imagine.

In John 14:1-3 we read: "Do not let your hearts be troubled. Trust in God; trust also in me. In my Father's house are many rooms; if it were not so, I would have told you. I am going there to prepare a place for you. And if I go and prepare a place for you, I will come back and take you to be with me that you also may be where I am." What an awesome promise!

I am thankful for the strength I was given yesterday. I enjoyed teaching my courses, enjoyed visits with students and conversations with colleagues. I was also grateful that I could spend a few precious moments with my aunt and cousins. Even through trials, God is good. These are the times we really take notice of who He is, and we recognize His abundant love for us.

Thank you God for your assurance of life, both here on earth and in eternal glory. Thank you for friends and neighbors and families that continue to do your work here on earth. Help us as we can only imagine, to forever worship You—on the good days and on the bummer days! Please be with the De Wit family today as they mourn the loss of their father and yet rejoice in his victory. Amen.

Friday, April 13, 2007 2:31 p.m.

Today I woke up exhausted again. Every day I hope that this fatigue will pass but so far it continues to plague me. I thought I knew what it meant to be tired. I've spent many a night getting just a few hours of sleep. I remember the nights before we left on vacation. In those days I was a neat freak so the house had to be spotless when we walked out the door. I always looked forward to walking back into a spotless house upon our return. I don't know why, because the only time it was clean was the time we were gone. By the time we walked in with all our dirty laundry and other stuff to be put away, you wouldn't have known the house had such a thorough cleaning.

There was often only a few hours of sleep the night before the first day of school too. I wanted the room to be perfect: name tags on the desks, new pencils sharpened and in the trays, bulletin boards full of color and meaningful messages, inspiring messages motivating the students, books and materials ready for instruction, and the room theme developed to perfection. Jerry has helped me hang "trees," put up a tent, construct a riding reading corner, and hang a lasso that encircled the biblical theme for the year. The best was the night we hung the tree. It was late in the evening and the temp was still around 100 degrees, and the humidity was even worse. As he lifted one of the ceiling tiles to attach a support for the tree, some (quite a bit) ceiling insulation came floating down. Oops—it looked as if he was tarred in white fluffy stuff. It was amazing the things Jerry got dragged into. And I must say most of it was done with a smile, well maybe not the hanging of the tree. Some of those nights were pretty short. But God blessed me with an unusual amount of energy. I sometimes felt a connection to the woman with the pitcher that never ran dry. It wasn't that I never got tired, but I always had energy to keep on going. Some of my friends gave me the nickname "The Midnight Rider" on our trips down to Cary, Mississippi. Others would occasionally call me the "Ever-Ready Bunny." I never thought too much of it; it was just a piece of who I was.

That piece of me has changed immensely over the past week. I've never in my life felt that drained. Every once in a while I think my energy level is going up, just to see it get zapped again. It's been difficult to motivate myself to get things done. I've never struggled with low energy before so this is something that has hit me both mentally and physically. I used to play a trick on myself. When I went to bed at night, I wouldn't look at the clock; that way when I tried to figure out how much sleep I'd had the night before, I couldn't come up with a number. I thought that not knowing made me feel less tired. It is amazing how much one's mental side can control the physical body. I thought I was pretty smart in developing this little trick. But it doesn't seem to have much use right now. I sleep no matter what time it is and what I have left undone. I'm so tired that I sleep more than I'm awake some days. And I can't do much about it.

When my family (and everyone who took their turn today), asked me how I was feeling, I ended up crying. Crying because I was frustrated, crying because I knew there was work I should have done, crying because of things I'm missing out on. So much for my plans, so much for my way of working things out. I'm not sure what God has planned for me. I've never understood the words of Jeremiah when he assures us that He has a plan and it will be a plan for my good. Right now that is hard for me to see, to understand, but I know that I can and will trust God for taking care of His plans.

After a big hug from Jerry and a steady dose of scripture, I feel better. It is amazing how God can lift your spirits, with or without energy, with or without a full head of hair!

These verses reminded me again of God's everlasting and solid love:

Find rest, O my soul, in God alone;
    my hope comes from him.
He alone is my rock and salvation;
    he is my fortress. I will not be shaken. (Psalm 62:5-6)

Sunday, April 15, 2007 1:17 a.m.

Yesterday was an exhausting day. It was the day of my Uncle Dutch's funeral. Our family has always been very close with the De Wit family so it was sad to see them mourn the loss of their husband, father and grandfather. The emotions of the day were broader though than the death of an uncle. As I watched from one of the last pews of the section saved for family members, I observed my family—aunts, uncles, mom and dad, cousins, and relatives from the other side. As Don De Wit beautifully sang "No More Night," I saw aunts and uncles mourn the spouses they had lost; I saw parents mourn children who had gone before them, and children mourn parents who were no longer on this earthly soil. Funerals seem to do that. They bring up memories of the past. For many of us it was a day of reflecting and checking on the order of our own lives. But the day wasn't only a day of sadness. There was a feeling of celebration. The songs, the scripture passages, the message, and the eulogy all showed evidence of the great hope and joy we have in our salvation. Knowing that Uncle Dutch and those who have gone before him, have received the gracious gift, the gift we celebrated last weekend, gave us a feeling of celebration. What peace that left with us.

I, too, was personally touched by the funeral and all that goes with it. It was a reminder to me of the frailty of life, the purpose of life, and the need to keep my eyes firmly fixed on my Heavenly Father. Right now Jesus is preparing a home for us. In John 14:1-4 John quotes Jesus: "Do not let your hearts be troubled. Trust in God; trust also in me. In my Father's house are many rooms; if it were not so, I would have told you. I am going there to prepare a place for you. And if I go and prepare a place for you, I will come back and take you to be with me that you also may be where I am. You know the way to the place where I am going." Because of Jesus' wonderful promise, all who believe in Him can have eternal life. I'm glad that we can sing with blessed assurance that Jesus is mine just as He has been for all those who have passed before us. What a blessing that we have been given a day to celebrate our risen Savior. Enjoy.

Monday, April 16, 2007 1:14 a.m.

Sunday morning followed a tough Saturday. Saturday was a day of exhaustion and Sunday was a day of frustration. My hair looked awful; I didn't want anyone to see it. I had spent a bunch of time trimming it on Saturday night. Well, to make a long story short, trimming bald spots is tough. I tried on my wig; it looked ridiculous on me (at least that's how I felt). Everything made me cry—Jerry looking at me, my looking at me, thinking about going out in public, everything. So I decided to stay home and watch our service on TV. I'm glad I did. Pastor Greg began his sermon talking about the effects of chemo treatments and how they wreak havoc on a person's body. Boy did I agree. That brought more emotions.

He then recited one of my favorite texts, one I know many of you love too—Isaiah 40:28-31: "God gives strength to the weary." Pastor Greg mentioned that many of the things we use need to be connected to some sort of power. You know what it's like—the electricity goes off and you feel as if your life has been cut off. You can't use the computer, the stove, the microwave, the TV, the radio. Without power all those objects are useless. It's like that for us in life too. We often cut ourselves off from our source of Power. We try to face our hard times alone; we slip away from studying His Word, we don't take time to pray; we drop out of Bible studies, and we don't take time to talk about spiritual things with our friends and family. Finding this power isn't about trusting our own faithfulness but instead it is about looking to our faithful One. Pastor Greg reminded us that this renewal is different than Paul's plea to have the thorn removed from him. It's a time when God transforms us through our trials. God works through us; He walks with us and strengthens us. It is a time when we have to "Turn our eyes upon Jesus. Look full in His wonderful face. And the things of earth will grow strangely dim, in the light of His glory and grace."

Pastor Greg finished with a great illustration. I hope he doesn't care that I share it but it was a great mental image for me. There was a missionary who lived in China. One day as he walked through the countryside, he observed a man pumping water from a well. What really surprised him was that the man never grew weary. He continued to pump without a break in his rhythm. This amazed the missionary. As he got closer he could see that what he thought was a real live man, was really a wooden cutout, a cutout whose arm was connected to the pump. The force of the Artesian water well was actually doing the work of pumping the water. We too have to keep our hand on the handle of God—connected to the power source, then He will direct; He will give strength; He will give power to the weak (that'd be me right now and maybe some of you who are reading this too). But with His power, I can soar like those eagles I've been seeing by the river.

Do you not know? Have you not heard?
The LORD is the everlasting God, the Creator of the ends of the earth. He will not grow tired or weary, and his understanding no one can fathom.
He gives strength to the weary and increases the power of the weak.
Even youths grow tired and weary. . . ;
but those who hope in the LORD will renew their strength.
They will soar on wings like eagles; they will run and not grow weary; they will walk and not be faint. (Isaiah 40:28-31)

Thanks for your continued support and prayers.

Tuesday, April 17, 2007 4:06 a.m.

Wasn't yesterday a beautiful day! I've been waiting for a day like this—warm temperatures, beautiful sun, and very little wind. Gorgeous! Days like that pick up my spirit. Yesterday was a lovely day, but it didn't take me very long into the day to realize that I didn't have to rely on the outside elements to "make my day." The warm greetings I received when I walked down the hall at work, the beautiful Gerber daisies (one of my favorite flowers) that I received from my friend Sandy, the offer from one of my students to donate her hair to "Locks of Love" for me, students eager to learn, enjoying my grandsons while watching my son-in-law coach his soccer team were all wonderful ways to enjoy the day. Is there anything better than hugs and kisses from your grandchildren? I was exhausted by the time I got home, but I was thankful for an enjoyable day. My emotions were much more in check; I had more energy and I'm getting used to my hair loss. I'm very thankful for good friends and family who continue to support us. Please continue to pray that the drugs are doing what they can do.

I'm feeling a little anxious about the perforation in the septum in my nose. I've had more pain and noticed more bleeding the past week. I also continue to struggle with fatigue. I'd love to have more energy but I know that this isn't possible, so please pray with me that I can learn how to use my time wisely and prioritize my activities. Every day is a blessing from God. I may not be able to do all that I would like to, but I'm thankful that I can continue to work and enjoy other activities. Most mornings

I wake up singing "This is the day that the Lord hath made, I will rejoice and be glad in it." Whether the day is sunny or cloudy, cold or warm, windy or calm, it's a day the Lord has given us to enjoy and use for His glory.

> This is the day the LORD has made;
>> let us rejoice and be glad in it. (Psalm 118:24)

Wednesday, April 18, 2007 6:51 a.m.

Good Morning,

Sabrina came to their house because she was told it was the Christians' house. She didn't live in the neighborhood but found herself there as she was literally walking her way across town. All she wanted was a ride. She asked but she didn't believe anyone would help her. That was the story that Megan told me last week. Mike and Megan (our daughter and son-in-law) live in a very poor section of Grand Rapids. They live in a community house that Calvin College has established. That means that they live in a house with five college students who, with Mike and Megan, work toward establishing relationships and helping people in the neighborhood. That's how the house got the name "The House of the Christians."

Sabrina is destitute. She has no job; her children are sometimes taken away from her; it is supposed that she makes money through prostitution; her boyfriend beats her into submission; and she doesn't appear to have much knowledge about God. It's hard to imagine a life like Sabrina's. I don't usually consider myself rich, but when I compare my life to Sabrina's, I admit that I am very rich. I'm rich because I own my house; I have a car; I have proper shoes for walking (although my colleagues might debate that), I have health insurance; I can go to a competent doctor; I have flowers in my living room and on my desk and much more. But more than that, I have a real relationship with Jesus Christ, not because of me, but because of Him.

Rob Bell in the segment called "Rich" from his Nooma series says, "Maybe you have this sense, you look around you and you have this sense that you don't have much because you see people who have even more. But it's a dangerous thing when we start to think the 'our' world is 'the' world. We're bombarded with all of these images of new models and the latest styles and after a while our stuff starts to seem kind of average, outdated, not-good-enough. That phrase, the God who richly provides us with everything, is true—all that we have is gift. Food–gift. Clothes–gift. Roof–gift. That breath that you just took—it's a gift."

In I Timothy 6:17-18 we read: "Command those who are rich in this present world not to be arrogant nor to put their hope in wealth, which is so uncertain, but to put their hope in God, who richly provides us with everything for our enjoyment. Command them to do good, to be rich in good deeds, and to be generous and willing to share." When I look at Sabrina, I realize my earthly treasures but even more than that I cherish my heavenly treasures—treasures I don't deserve but have been given by God. And if I truly appreciate those treasures, what do I do to thank God? It isn't an easy question. Oh, we can give by going to church, reading the Bible, and praying. Those are the kinds of answers I would often receive from my second and fifth graders, but I'm afraid that's an answer I give too. If I consider myself rich, then I have to consider the question, "What can I give?" What can I do to be more generous? I've learned many lessons from those around me who have showered me with generosity the past few months. Many have truly given—from their heart. You've asked the question.

Rob Bell concludes his message by saying, "May you come to see that you are rich. And may you do what Jesus says, may you step into your divine responsibility to give, and when you do, may you take hold of the life that is truly life." Just as Mike and Megan are showing Christ to Sabrina, I hope I can find the Sabrinas around me and reach out to them. In the next verse of I Timothy 6 we read: "In this way they will lay up treasures for themselves as a firm foundation for the coming age, so they may take hold of the life that is truly life" (vs. 19). In His Love.

Thursday, April 19, 2007 8:15 a.m.

Yesterday was an exciting day. Earlier this school year the library staff asked if I would be willing to be photographed for a poster that would go up in the library to promote reading. They began this project last year and hope to continue it in the years to come. I chose a children's book that told the story of a Laotian family coming to America, very similar to how Sou's family (our son-in-law) came here. Because the book was for children, I asked if my oldest three grandchildren could be on the picture with me. The picture is very similar to the picture on the cover of the CaringBridge page. Yesterday was the unveiling. Some of my family members were there, some colleagues, a few students, and the library

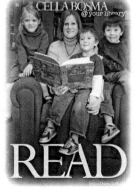

staff. Sheryl Taylor, the head librarian, (sorry Sheryl, I can't think of a better title right now) talked a little about the purpose behind the posters and then announced that the fines collected during this week, National Library Week, were going to be given to the Susan B. Komen Breast Cancer Foundation in honor of me. Another humbling experience. (Sheryl and I had a little trouble getting through our speeches.) Sheryl also had pink wrist bands and ribbons to hand out this week as a visual reminder of breast cancer. The library staff has been particularly supportive during my journey the past few months. They prepared a tasty basket of food very early on, donated a cart with garden equipment for the auction, sent numerous notes of encouragement, provided lots of hugs, and now have supported a research foundation. Thank you library staff for all you have done. You have encouraged me in many ways.

I was initially very surprised to be asked to be on the READ poster and I still am. At the time I was asked to participate in the poster project I had no idea of what would be going on in my life on April 19, 2007. None of us knew how different life would be in a few short months. Yes-

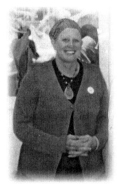

terday was a good reminder to me that the future is unknown. It reminded me how quickly things can change and how important it is to walk each day as an important day. I don't want to sound morbid, but for any of us, we don't know what tomorrow will bring. James 4:13-17 reminds us: "Now listen, you who say, 'Today or tomorrow we will go to this or that city' . . . . Why, you do not even know what will happen tomorrow. What is your life? You are a mist that appears for a little while and then vanishes . . . . Anyone, then, who knows the good he ought to do and doesn't do it, sins." The future is in God's hands. What a reminder to live for God today.

In a few minutes I'm leaving to meet Mindy who will take me for another round of chemo. This will be the first of three in the second series. I've been extremely fatigued again the past few days. I think the library unveiling yesterday must have worn me out. With the exception of about an hour break around 6:00, I slept from 3:00 p.m. until this morning. I just couldn't get out of the tired mode. I feel better this morning and am praying that nothing in the blood tests will delay my treatments. It should be a lovely day for a drive to Sioux Falls. I love the sun. Enjoy your day.

Friday, April 20, 2007 1:58 a.m.

Good Morning,

(Yes, I am up late. Once the Benadryl wears off, the drug that hypes me up kicks in.)

When a chemo patient shows up for treatment, each one longs to hear, "Your counts look good." Those words were like music to my ears yesterday when Dr. Krie came into the exam room and said them to me. I think all cancer patients feel anxious as they await the results of the blood tests. If your counts are too low, you are sent home to wait until the next week to see if they come up. I complained much about the white cell booster, but it must have done its job because my white cell count was very high. Dr. Krie doesn't think she'll give me the shot again because it caused much pain and extreme fatigue so I hope my white count can stay up. The treatment today went well. I tolerated the drugs well and again slept soundly after the Benadryl. I'm thankful that so far I haven't experienced the side effects that are associated with the drugs.

I appreciate my visits with Dr. Krie. She is knowledgeable, compassionate, and I enjoy visiting with her. She is very concerned about how I feel and what is happening in my life. But after our visits I always leave with some uncertainty, and I really feel in need of prayers. She always reminds me that metastasized cancer means that I'll be on chemo for a long time, if not forever. That scares me but I continue to hang on to the hope of healing. Last night I looked at all the references to healing in the concordance of the Bible and once again was reminded of the healing power of God. God is a mighty God, a God who can conquer cancer or any other disease. I know I've quoted these verses before but today they are again very meaningful to me.

"May the God of hope fill you with all joy and peace as you trust in him, so that you may overflow with hope by the power of the Holy Spirit" (Romans 15:13).

"But now, Lord, what do I look for? My hope is in you" (Psalm 39:7).

Orison Swett Marden once said: "There is no medicine like hope, no incentive so great, and no tonic so powerful as expectation of something better tomorrow."

So many of you have told me that you are praying for complete healing—that adds to my feeling of hope. Thank you for giving that to me.

I would like to add a note of encouragement to women who read this entry. Please take time for a yearly checkup. I know—it takes time; it isn't always pleasant; it can even be scary. Those are some of the reasons

I gave for putting off going in for my checkup. But I truly believe that God gives us these opportunities in order to detect cancer early. If I could change one thing, it would be to have had my recheck quicker. I know I'm on the journey planned for me, but it could be different for you. So please, take the time to make an appointment; it could make a difference in your life.

Saturday, April 21, 2007 1:49 a.m.

Good Saturday Morning,

Amira is our only granddaughter. She is a special delight. She has a zest for life like none other! She is a very perceptive little girl and loves to share her thoughts. This week Megan was helping the preschool teacher plan some activities to help broaden the cultural awareness of the students. Miss Lorna asked Megan to share some Nigerian traditions with the students. She decided to share a recipe, explain the naming ceremony that is very common in Nigerian families, make an art activity, practice carrying things on their heads, and do baby wraps. Megan cut some pieces of cloth big enough for the preschoolers to use to tie their favorite stuffed animals to their backs just like the moms do in Nigeria. Megan explained her plans to Amira and then asked her if she thought the students would like these activities. Amira looked at Megan and said, "Oh Mom, they'll be delighted." Isn't it great to see how easily children are delighted! To delight means to experience great joy and pleasure. It made me wonder how often we take time to delight in our wonderful God and His created world.

How often do we take time to delight in His people? Do we look for the good qualities of others or is it easier to pick them apart? Do we look for the potential of others or do we write them off for who they are today? How often do you take time to delight in His creation? Do you take time to see the budding trees and the blooming flowers? Do you see them as marvelous productions of nature? Do you see the beautiful colors of creation as a representation of God's diversity?

And here is the big question: How often do we take time to delight in the Lord? To delight in the Lord, we have to know Him. When we learn about Him we see His great love for us and it gives us delight. It also helps us commit ourselves to the Lord. The NIV commentary on Psalm 37:4-5 reads: "To commit ourselves to the Lord means to trust in him, believing that he can care for us better than we can ourselves. We should be willing to wait patiently for him to work out what is best for us." Those words really spoke to me. I need to work on patience as I wait for Him to work out His plans for me. I'm going to try to take more time to delight in God's world. I'm sure I'll be amazed!

> Delight yourself in the Lord
>> and he will give you the desires of your heart.
> Commit your way to the Lord;
>> trust in him and he will do this:
> He will make your righteousness shine like the dawn,
>> the justice of your cause like the noonday sun.
> Be still before the LORD and wait patiently for him . . . .
> (Psalm 37:4-7a)

Today was a great day. I felt good, enjoyed teaching, loved the warm weather, and had the opportunity to enjoy helping my young friend Jaleesa prepare for her prom. What fun it was to see a beautiful young girl, both inside and out, get ready for her exciting night. It almost made me wish I were young again—almost.

Monday, April 23, 2007 12:28 a.m.

Jerry is a real trooper. He displayed the ultimate demonstration of love last Friday night. He shaved off the last of my hair—there were just small bunches left. I had a hard time deciding to bite the bullet and shave it all off, but late Friday I looked in the mirror and decided it had to go. I thought about calling someone to help me but didn't want to put anyone through this so I started shaving. It wasn't nearly as bad as I thought it would be. I couldn't reach the back of my head well, so when Jerry came home, he patiently and carefully buzzed off the last few strands. Besides having to ask him occasionally not to bump the shaver against my very tender head, it went well. We laughed at how we thought this was something that would be happening to Jerry, not to me. He's been balding a little over the past few years, but suddenly he has much more hair than I! I was surprised how easy it was to actually cut off the last of my hair. I thought I might feel a real loss but it hasn't been emotional at all. I think God has led me through tiny steps to help prepare me. Two weeks ago this might have been traumatic, but after looking at bald spots and continuing to see hair fall out, it was actually a relief to be finished with it.

At this time I've decided not to wear my wig. It makes me feel unnatural and it feels as if I've got a sign on that says, "Bald woman." I've decided to wear scarves and hats instead. It's amazing how many women have come up to me in the last week and have told me that they noticed my scarf or hat and wonder if I'm going through chemo. All have been survivors and have offered encouragement. What a blessing these women have been to me! This experience has made me wonder about the times I've kept my burdens to myself. I don't want people to know about my heartaches or the problems in my life so I hide them. I carry the burden alone. I live in a small community and sometimes I'm worried that my concerns will turn to town gossip so I give up the opportunity to feel and experience the love of the community.

In Galatians 6:2 we read: "Carry each other's burdens, and in this way you will fulfill the law of Christ." Matthew 11:28-30 assures us that Jesus takes our burdens upon Himself and frees us from them. If we take our burdens to Him, He promises us love, healing, and peace with God: "Come to me, all you who are weary and burdened, and I will give you rest. Take my yoke upon you and learn from me, for I am gentle and humble in heart, and you will find rest for your souls. For my yoke is easy and my burden is light." So, if you are carrying a burden in your heart, consider sharing it. God can take that burden away. He can also use people to help you carry your burden. Or, if you see someone with a burden, reach out and help to relieve their load.

What a friend we have in Jesus, all our sins and griefs to bear!
What a privilege to carry everything to God in prayer.
Oh, what peace we often forfeit, oh, what needless pain we bear,
All because we do not carry everything to God in prayer.

Tuesday, April 24, 2007 8:09 a.m.

Sunday evening as I walked on the sidewalk that leads to our church, I tried to avoid all the brown gunk on the sidewalk. It looked disgusting and I didn't want it on my shoes. At first I wasn't sure what the brown stuff was but when I looked around, especially up, I figured out I was walking on the shells that had fallen off the branches of the trees that grace the lawn of our church property. The coverings fell off as the leaf buds began to swell and push off the protective coverings, allowing the new leaves to push forward. The branches are now filled with green tips that will soon develop into lush green-filled branches. The beauty didn't just happen. First, the cold weather had to disappear—the coming out of the leaves is a response to temperature change. The change in the temperature causes a hormonal release in the tree and that triggers the sprouting of leaves. This allows for photosynthesis to begin so the plant can carry on total life functions again.

Isn't that exactly like our Christian life? We need the power of the Son to start the process. When Jesus Christ becomes that power in our life, it changes. We begin to blossom for Him. Just as the shells fell off the branches and left yucky residue, so it is with sin. When we begin to focus on Jesus Christ, the sin in our life begins to drop off. That doesn't mean that we become sinless, but it does become evident, just like the green budding on the trees, that we are following what Christ modeled for us in life. This should affect the way we live each day—our work, worship, and play. It influences our decisions, the way we treat others, and what we think, say and do. As we read in Romans 6:8-14: "Now if we died with Christ, we believe that we will also live with him. For we know that since Christ was raised from the dead, he cannot die again; death no longer has mastery over him. The death he died, he died to sin once for all; but the life he lives, he lives to God. In the same way, count yourselves dead to sin but alive to God in Christ Jesus. Therefore do not let sin reign in your mortal body so that you obey its evil desires . . . rather offer yourselves to God, as those who have been brought from death to life; and offer the parts of your body to him as instruments of righteousness. For sin shall not be your master, because you are not under law, but under grace."

Like the gunk on the sidewalk, sin is disgusting. Just as I tried to avoid that gunk as I was walking to church, I have to try to avoid the sin that so easily permeates my life. Only by looking to the Son will I have the power to accomplish this. Where will you see the buds of green in your life?

Tuesday, April 24, 2007 11:28 p.m.

My head is causing me some problems—on the outside. I have a rash over most of it. It looks awful but worse than that, it hurts. I've tried a bunch of different creams and lotions but nothing seems to work. I'm trying not to scratch my head, but I've never been good at self-control when it comes to an itch. A bald head is not too attractive but a bald head with red spots—that just doesn't count as beauty. But hey, even without hair I think I look better than this madam. (I'll have to work on getting the picture tomorrow. It wouldn't transfer when I was updating. It's worth seeing.) But then I guess beauty is in the eye of the beholder. But even more importantly, beauty is only skin deep. It isn't the outside that counts but the inside, right? All my life I've been told that, but sometimes, especially when I look into the mirror today, it is hard to believe. As much as I don't like it, I must admit that I do get caught up in what I can see and not what's on the inside. In our culture today we get the message that outward beauty is what counts. It's all about buying this or that product that is going to make you beautiful. This cream will take away the wrinkles from around your eyes; this product will firm up your thighs (I'm always interested in this one), another will help you lose ten pounds in three days. Unfortunately none of these quick fixes really work. And they aren't the most important thing in life anyway.

In I Samuel 16:7 we read: "But the LORD said to Samuel, 'Do not consider his appearance or his height, for I have rejected him. The LORD does not look at the things man looks at. Man looks at the outward appearance, but the LORD looks at the heart.'" God looks at our character, not our appearance. God is the only one who can see what's inside and that's what is important. Many of us spend hours maintaining our outward appearance, but how much time do we spend developing our inner character? Everyone can see my bald head with spots, but only God can know what my heart really looks like. I need to look at what steps I'm taking to improve my attitude.

Thanks again for all the cards, words of encouragement, and prayers. Every day I'm amazed at those of you who take time to e-mail me, check my website, write in my CaringBridge site, and send things through snail mail. Besides my hurting scalp, I'm again experiencing fatigue. I have only a week and a half of classes left, and I'm praying that I can keep up my energy so I can finish out the year strong. Please pray with me. Thank you.

Thursday, April 26, 2007 9:06 a.m.

Hello everyone,

Mom was too tired to write in the journal last night and she had to leave early this morning for her treatment so she will write later on. Please continue to pray for her that her blood counts are good so that she can have her treatment today. Thank you all for your prayers; we can definitely feel them! Mindy

Friday, April 27, 2007 1:04 a.m.

God's grace. What a wonderful gift! I am continually blessed by His grace.

Yesterday my friend Lorna and I left for my treatment in Sioux Falls at around 7:30 a.m. I was nervous. What if the doctor found my counts low? I wondered if the sores on my head were caused by the chemo and if that would hinder my treatment. We arrived at the center around 9:00. I didn't have to see Dr. Krie today so I was sent to the infusion room as soon as we arrived. Lisa drew blood from my port and sent it to the lab and then the wait began. During the wait time, most of the staff, including Dr. Krie, came to check my head. It was a hot topic of conversation. Dr. Krie was worried that the redness was due to the treatments and wondered if we should stop the treatments for a week. I nearly got on my knees to beg her to reconsider. I was sure it was due to the abrasiveness of the razor that I used on my head when I shaved off my hair. The timing seemed to coincide—I shaved my head on Friday and my head began to hurt on Saturday. After some talking, she decided to go ahead with chemo if my counts were good and then told me to watch the redness and spots on my head. That was one hurdle. More waiting.

Finally I saw Lisa walk from the nurses' area with a bag of fluid in her hand and I knew my counts were okay. Actually my white count was excellent and so was my blood pressure! That was another hurdle. God's grace. My Sioux Falls friend Lorna, who is also receiving cancer treatment, came over to say hello before she went into her doctor's appointment because she knew I would be asleep by the time she got into the infusion room. She was right; the next time I saw her she was sitting a few chairs away from me receiving her chemo and my treatment was finished. It was good to talk to her again. God's grace.

My chemo treatment again went very well. I didn't have any negative reactions. Another hurdle and some more of God's grace. I was even awake enough after my treatment to enjoy lunch with my Sanborn Lorna and my sister Marcia. God's grace again. In the past few days, many people have shown me the grace that can only come from God. There was the funny card I found under my door, the encouraging conversations with colleagues, unexpected messages from relatives and from new and old friends and acquaintances, encouragement from students, some inspiring e-mails, CaringBridge entries, and support from my family. Jerry continues to help with the cooking, Josh helps with daily tasks around the house, and the girls always call to see how I'm doing.

Pastor Rod Gorter, the campus pastor from Dordt, often called me after my surgery. In one of our conversations, he reminded me that no matter what—no matter who I am, what I've done, or how I've messed up, God's grace is always there for me. I don't have to earn it. I don't have to work for it. I just have to accept it. The things that happened to me today didn't happen because of who I am but because of who God is. What a comfort! What a God! God's grace was there for me today as it has been in the past and will be in the future. God has shown His free and unmerited favor for me. "For all have sinned and fall short of the glory of God, and are justified freely by his grace through the redemption that came by Jesus Christ" (Romans 3:23-24).

Each day I realize that God's grace is sufficient for me. In II Corinthians 12:9 Paul says, "My grace is sufficient for you, for my power is made perfect in weakness."

Just to let you know: I'm not sure how many of you prayed, but your prayers must have been powerful. Toward late afternoon I noticed that my head was itching less, and by the time I got home it had almost stopped inching. I still have a rash, but I don't think my head is as red. There may have been some medicine in the pre-drugs that helped with the healing, but I don't discount the prayers that were lifted up. Dr. Krie put me on an antibiotic for ten days which should continue to help with the healing. I'm very thankful for your prayers and for the relief of pain.

Saturday, April 28, 2007 8:38 a.m.

Good Morning,

We used to own a vehicle that had this warning written on the bottom of the rear view mirror—Caution, objects may be closer than they appear. I'm not good at details, so I didn't take notice of this little warning until I nearly ran a car off the road. That got my attention (and some honks and dirty looks too). From then on I tried to pay attention to those tiny words and watch for the false image it created. I've found this to be true in my life too. I'm pretty good at giving a false image. When you talk to me, I may appear to have my life under control. I can fake a pretty good smile and talk a pretty line but the truth is plain and simple: I hate cancer. Today is one of those days that I can't get it out of my mind. I hate it. I hate what it has done to my body; I hate what it has done to my head. I can't say I hate how it makes me feel because it is such a silent disease, but I do hate how the drugs have made me feel. I hate always feeling fatigued. I hate that it has put an extra burden on my colleagues. I hate all the involvement in church that I've had to give up, and I hate how it makes me feel less of a wife, mother, and grandmother.

There, I feel a little better. Sometimes you have to get it out of your system. God has treated us with a beautiful day today; the sun is shining brilliantly and there is the promise of warmth. My neighbor Phyllis noticed that over the winter my hydrangeas died so she brought over a beautiful purple-headed flower and set it by my glass back door. I again received cards and messages from unexpected people and from some very special friends; they brought pure joy. Megan called to say that a woman in her church who had been diagnosed with the same kind of cancer as I, only she had more spots on her lungs, was just told that she is cancer free for now; what hope. God has given me many words of instruction that give me hope, and yet I ignore them. Sometimes it's easier for me to wallow in my sorrow than to keep my eye on the hope that is all around me. Like the words on the rear view mirror, I can see them but when I don't follow the instructions, I get into trouble.

I have these promises from God:

Philippians 4:7: "And the peace of God, which transcends all understanding, will guard your hearts and your minds in Christ Jesus." Psalm 30:5: "Weeping may remain for a night, but rejoicing comes in the morning." Matthew 11:28-29: Jesus said, "Come to me, all you who are weary and burdened, and I will give you rest. Take my yoke upon you and learn from me, for I am gentle and humble in heart, and you will find rest for your souls."

Charles Spurgeon wrote, "There is no cry so good as that which comes from the bottom of the mountains; no prayer half so hearty as that which comes up from the depths of the soul through deep trials and afflictions. For they bring us to God and we are happier; for nearness to God is happiness."

I have promises from people:

I hear and see it all around me. I never go one day without people assuring me that they are praying for me. What astonishment! I can't say thanks enough. I know this sense of despair can only last a little while if I keep my eyes on Jesus and if I entrust this time to God. I can also take my cue from the world around me—-His nature and His people. Today I'm praying that I can concentrate on the joys that abound in my life and move past the frustrations with which I began. I'm going to fight the feelings. I think I'll make a sign that says: Danger: feelings are closer than they look. But I'll add: Look to Jesus!

Monday, April 30, 2007 6:59 a.m.

Good Morning,

Yesterday was a wonderful but exhausting day. I'm leaving soon for school, my last full week of teaching. I'll post something later this morning. Have a good day.

Monday, April 30, 2007 1:57 p.m.

To be honest I was a little afraid of sharing my true thoughts in my journal last Saturday, but I have learned that when I verbalize my needs, God opens up avenues to encourage me. I've also learned that people are great at being specific in their prayers when they know of specific needs, so I left myself quite vulnerable and opened my heart. I think it was a

God thing. Along with thoughtful and specific prayers, I received many blessings. God's people are surely gifted and creative in knowing how to provide encouragement.

One act of kindness that really touched me came unexpectedly. A woman whom a few months ago I would have considered an acquaintance but now consider a friend, came over after reading my journal entry with a wild berry smoothie, a favorite of mine. She also showed me a sanctuary that she used when she was going through chemo treatments and invited me to use it any time I felt the need. It's a tranquil place not far from my house, a place where I can reflect and meditate. It was a wonderful and unexpected gift. If there is one thing I have learned through this experience it's that gifts are not always material. Tangible things are nice and very much appreciated, but so are those unexpected gifts like words and hugs and places of solace. Yesterday I had the opportunity to talk to many people whom I haven't seen in a long while. Those conversations were gifts too. Thanks to all of you who have "gifted" me in so many ways. I'm going to work on my creativity. I'm still struggling with the rash on my head. It does seem to be getting some better but it still itches. I had more energy over the past few days but I did come home early today to catch a nap so I hope I can get some work done later today. Blessings to all of you.

MAY/JUNE 2007

Tuesday, May 1, 2007 7:39 a.m.

Good Morning,

A good friend of mine is serving with the Peace Corps in Camaroon. When Kate was a senior at Dordt College, she and I went with a mission team to Nicaragua. Kate and I spent time together hanging in the coffee bean trees, picking the red beans as we struggled to avoid falling out of the trees and down the steep hills. Even though we had to work hard to fight the pull of gravity, pick the beans, and get them into the bags tied around our waist, we were still able to have great conversations. We talked about life as it was and life in the future.

In a recent e-mail, Kate talked about her work in Africa. She's just recently come to realize that she's "hit the wall" in her work over there. If you're a runner, you probably know what it's like to "hit the wall." It's the point where you feel as if you are standing still, like your legs are moving in slow motion, and you just can't go any more. It happens when you are physically, mentally, and emotionally exhausted. It's the point where you can't see the finish line and even if you could, the hard work of getting there doesn't seem worth it. Any good track coach will tell you that if you can push past the wall, you can finish the race strong. You may need a drink of water or a shot of gel to give you that final burst of energy, but you'll have the strength to complete the race. Kate is looking for ways to overcome her exhaustion and lack of energy. It won't come in the way of food but rather in refocusing and looking to God for guidance. I know Kate, and I'm confident she'll get past her wall and finish strong.

In our Christian life we sometimes "hit the wall" too. For some reason we reach a point in our life where we find following God's will for our life tough. We become physically, mentally, emotionally, and spiritually tired. We feel as if it's too much work to live stewardly; we give up on loving our neighbor; we lose our desire to live right. We give up. It just seems like too much effort and work. We somehow can't see the finish line. Just as we may need an extra boost of liquid when running a long foot-race, we also need an extra boost in our spiritual life. We need continual spiritual refocusing to help us continue the race. Sometimes this refreshment comes through worship, prayer, a devotional, a conversation with another Christian, or reflection on a Bible passage. If we want to finish the race strong, it's important that we look for ways to be refreshed.

For instance:

Acts 20:24: "However, I consider my life worth nothing to me, if only I may finish the race and complete the task the Lord Jesus has given me."

I Corinthians 9:24-25:"Do you not know that in a race all the runners run, but only one gets the prize? Run in such a way as to get the prize. Everyone who competes in the games goes into strict training. They do it to get a crown that will not last; but we do it to get a crown that will last forever."

Just to let you know: My head rash seems a little better. Last night I found information on the Internet that suggested using a dusting of corn starch to relieve the itching. So late last night I threw some corn starch on my head. It didn't reap instant results but it doesn't seem that it can hurt my head so I may continue with the corn starch for a while longer. I had a burst of energy last night. It felt good! I went for a walk and then began working on a dinner that I am preparing for one of my classes on Wednesday. As I said, it felt good—so good to be at almost a normal energy level once again. Have a good day and thanks for all you've done.

Wednesday, May 2, 2007 8:45 a.m.

Good Morning,

Since Monday afternoon I have been blessed with renewed energy. I have felt almost normal except for a few itches and an occasional headache. I'm looking forward to today and need an extra boost of energy to complete all I have planned. Today I'm taking treats to school in appreciation for all the help and support the librarians have given me throughout this semester and every semester. My Applied Education Psych class is coming over for dinner tonight. That would have been a normal day last semester, but it is quite an accomplishment for me right now. I'm very thankful for the extra energy.

Now that I've brought up my students, I want to share something with you that I read to one of my classes last week. I found this parable in Chuck Swindoll's book *Growing Strong in the Seasons of Life*.

"A Rabbit on the Swim Team"

Once upon a time the animals decided they should do something meaningful to meet the problems of the new world. So they organized a school.

They adopted an activity curriculum of running, climbing,

swimming, and flying. To make it easier to administer the curriculum, all the animals took all the subjects.

The *duck* was excellent in swimming; in fact, better than his instructor. But he made only passing grades in flying, and was very poor in running. Since he was slow in running, he had to drop swimming and stay after school to practice running. This caused his web feet to be badly worn, so that he was only average in swimming. But average was quite acceptable, so nobody worried about that—except the *duck.*

The *rabbit* started at the top of his class in running, but developed a nervous twitch in his leg muscles because of so much make-up work in swimming.

The *squirrel* was excellent in climbing, but he encountered constant frustration in flying class because his teacher made him start from the ground up instead of from the treetop down. He developed "charley horses" from overexertion, and so only got a C in climbing and a D in running.

The *eagle* was a problem child and was severely disciplined for being a non-conformist. In climbing classes he beat all the others to the top of the tree but insisted on using his own way to get there . . .

The reason I read this parable to my students is that I want each of them to be aware that they will teach a wide variety of students. But it's like that for you and me too—we come into contact with a wide variety of characteristics in the people we meet—our families, our coworkers, our neighbors, our fellow church members. Like the animals in the parable, each of them has been blessed with a wide variety of gifts and abilities. Sometimes we make the mistake of trying to make everyone the same. We expect the same things out of different people. And sometimes we make the mistake of thinking that everyone should be like us! God wants each of us to be ourselves. He wants us to use our gifts to bless his kingdom. I hope you will take time to read I Corinthians 12. It gives a great explanation of how God can use all of us. And remember—there is plenty of room in the forest. Be yourself and serve God the way He intended you to and let others serve Him as they were intended to.

Thursday, May 3, 2007 5:18 a.m.

Good Morning,

I was exhausted. Absolutely and terribly exhausted but it was a good exhaustion. This exhaustion was different from the fatigue I've been experiencing the past month. It was due to what seemed like a hundred trips up and down the steps to the fridge in the garage, bringing food up and down for the dinner with my students. I was finally finished for the night. Dinner with my students was over and I had every dish and pan washed and put away. Even though I was tired, I had a great feeling of satisfaction. Isn't that what hard work does? It's been a long time since I was actually tired from hard work. I enjoyed the planning, the preparation, the meal and, yes, even the cleanup. I'm thankful for the renewed energy that allowed me to enjoy the year-end celebration with my students. We enjoyed our meal, chatting as we ate fresh spinach, lasagna, and death by chocolate (the dessert). Usually I'm the one doing most of the talking, but this time I was the listener. The students talked about their future plans. It was fun to hear them energetically tell about their summer plans, upcoming weddings, and student teaching assignments. I learned a lot about my students.

Listening isn't something we're very good at. In today's society we are more apt to talk than to listen. In fact, often when we listen we are planning what we are going to say next. That's really not listening. In Psalm 46:10 we are instructed to "Be still, and know." This instruction is given so that we can know God better, but it's good instruction for us in getting to know others better too. I hope you take time today to listen; listen intently so you can know someone else better.

"He who answers before listening—that is his folly and his shame" (Proverbs 18:13).

Mike's (my son-in-law) mother is taking me for treatments today. I'm feeling so good that I am confident my blood work will test well enough for me to receive the treatment. I'm thankful for the return to some normalcy in my energy level. I'm also thankful for all of you who continue to encourage and support me. This is my last treatment in my second series. One more series to go and then a PET scan. If you will, please continue to pray that the drugs are doing what they have been proven to do. Cella

Friday, May 4, 2007 5:39 a.m.

Good Day,

Some days I fall into the trap of feeling sorry for myself. Job 10 tells of Job's despair with God's dealings and describes his fall into self-pity. The footnote for this verse found in the NIV Bible reads: "When we face baffling affliction, our pain lures us toward feeling sorry for ourselves. At that point we are only one step from self-righteousness, where we keep track of life's injustices and say, 'Look what happened to me; how unfair it is!' We may feel like blaming God. Remember that life's trials, whether allowed by God or sent by God, can be the means for development and refinement. When facing trials, ask, 'What can I learn and how can I grow?' rather than 'Who did this to me and how can I get out of it?'" What have I learned?

I've learned to develop my problem-solving skills. In the last two weeks I've had to figure how to lie in a supine position (the best position for sleeping) and yet position myself to avoid the pain caused by the pressure of lying on my rash. Over the past two weeks, I've discovered that by tilting a little on my left side and bending my hips at a 33 degree angle with my knees and feet at 90 degree angles, putting the thumb of my right hand just to the inside of my ear and my fingers on the bald spot just behind my ear, I can sleep comfortably. How about that for being creative?

Seriously though, I have learned much over the past few months. Along with a whole new medical vocabulary, I've learned that God shows Himself through a bazillion (maybe that's a little exaggeration) caring medical people who work in many different medical facilities. Yesterday, again, I was the recipient of the great love of my doctor, her staff, and the nurses in the infusion room. As I was reclining in the long line of infusion room chairs with the drugs dripping into my port, Dan, the male nurse, offered a prayer over the intercom system for National Prayer Day. I must be honest and say that I don't remember much of the prayer because the Benadryl was doing its thing, but I was comforted to know that the people who are taking care of me believe and love the same God that I love and believe in. And as you know, because you've been a part of this, I've also learned about the great ways people serve God. And all of this *has* brought me closer to God. I've been reminded again and again that God does not forsake nor leave me. I've learned that He continues to love me even when I question and doubt. I've learned how to find peace in an unrestful situation.

How can I grow? I have many ways to grow, spiritually that is. (Please, no jokes about the physical.) Each day I continue to better understand who God is. I'm learning how to "see" Him all around me. I hope, too, that I am growing in ways to serve Him. And I hope that I can grow in asking when, what, and how, instead of who and why.

I'm thankful for this great big, beautiful God who keeps me in the palm of His hand each and every day. I can grow by reading these passages: Job 10:1: "I loathe my very life; therefore I will give free rein to my complaint and speak out in the bitterness of my soul." In Job 42 Job replies to God's questions in chapter 38: "I know that you can do all things; no plan of yours can be thwarted." Assurance for growth comes from Philippians 1:6: " . . . being confident of this, that he who began a good work in you will carry it on to completion until the day of Christ Jesus."

Saturday, May 5, 2007 1:07 a.m.

Good Morning,

I was reminded yesterday that I didn't tell you about my good visit with Dr. Krie. It was a very encouraging visit. She was extremely happy with my counts. My hemoglobin was excellent, as was my red blood-cell count. My blood pressure was up a little and my white count was down but neither was in the danger zone. I received both Avastin and Paxil and those treatments went very well. The rash on my head is starting to disappear and she gave me a prescription for a gel to apply to see if we can get rid of it completely. At my appointment I told Dr. Krie that I had very minimal tingling of my hands and feet, a side effect that will eventually make me quit this treatment. Well, last night I had the beginning of the pain. My fingers don't tingle too much but my feet are really hurting. Dr. Krie is hoping that having two weeks off will help decrease the pain. She's actually hoping that I can take three more series of these drugs before she changes to another drug. We talked about what will happen after the third series. Right now I'm looking at waiting a week or two after the third series to have a scan. She feels this will give the most accurate reading. Dr. Krie said I could have either a PET or CT scan and since the CT "juice" made me feel really sick last time, she suggested we try the PET. The PET scan doesn't give us numbers like a CT scan but it is accurate in telling if the tumor has shrunk. I wasn't given a white cell booster after this series so Dr. Krie encouraged me to avoid others who are sick. She felt the reaction I had to the shot wasn't worth it. So now we hope that my body will reproduce its own white blood cells during the two weeks off. I'm thankful that I've responded well to the drugs so far. My energy level has been much better this week. It's great to be able to put in a full day's work once again.

One of the things I'm again reminded of is the importance of trusting God. When I look back on my life, I see how often I've trusted in myself. I know that the only way I'm going to make it through this experience is to turn my trust from myself to God. As the treatments take a toll on my body, I pray that my soul will retain its child-like trust, a trust that clings to the simple promise of salvation through the blood of Jesus

Christ. Each of us, as we experience trials in life, stumble in our broken-ness to the Savior, in knowing that He is the only one who can renew and restore us. One thing I can be sure of is this—that the Master will not turn me away. He promises to gather me in His arms and assures me of His love and care. He promises that to you too:

> "Surely God is my salvation;
>   I will trust and not be afraid.
> The LORD, the LORD, is my strength and my song;
>   he has become my salvation."
> With joy you will draw water
>   from the wells of salvation. (Isaiah 12:2-3)

> My comfort in my suffering is this:
> Your promise preserves my life. (Psalm 119:50)

Monday, May 7, 2007 8:19 a.m.

Just to let you know: I'm going to add a short piece to my journal this morning. I've once again been hit with extreme fatigue. Saturday I spent most of the day sleeping. Kenzie and Paige, two wonderful little friends of mine, brought over some beautiful Gerber daisies in the af-ternoon and invited us over for supper. We had a wonderful time and it did feel good to get up for a while. On Sunday I played for the morning service. I loved playing for the service, especially since Cath and Michele played their instruments with me, but it definitely zapped my energy. We went to Nate and Mary Beth's house for a delicious lunch and then I again spent the rest of the day sleeping. I'm hoping I'll get some energy back today. Thanks for keeping me in your prayers.

Tuesday, May 8, 2007 8:25 a.m.

Fatigue has been a big part of my life the past few days. I've spent a lot of time on the couch catching as much sleep as I could. Some-times I couldn't sleep but being too tired to get up, I often gazed out of our living room windows. Since we live in a split-level house, the only thing I could see were the trees that surround our house. Those trees were a lesson to me. From my position on the couch I could see a red maple, some locust trees, a mulberry, and an evergreen. All were in different stages of budding. The evergreen, of course, in its ever green stage, looked the same now as it did all winter. The red maple's leaves are out and it looks quite different from a month ago. The locust trees are almost fully developed and the mulberry leaves are only about half open. As I lay there, the trees reminded me of the Christian life. For one, the trees reminded me of the lives of people in God's kingdom. Each of us is in a different stage. Some "open" early and have lived a long life serving God. Some are new believers and are just coming to know God. But all have life and beauty and purpose in His kingdom. The budding trees also reminded me of my life. There are times when I feel close to God, a time I'm in full bloom, a time when I feel connected to God. I also experience times when I doubt God, when I feel alienated from Him, a time when I'm searching. Keeping an eye on each stage is important. When we feel the disconnect, when we struggle to know and believe in God, we can be assured that the everlasting Father, the evergreen tree, is always there for us. He is there to help us as we develop and bloom. I'm reminded of Ken Miedema's "The Tree Song":

I saw a tree by the riverside one day as I walked along.
Straight as an arrow pointing to the sky growing tall and strong.
"How do you grow so tall and strong?" I said to the riverside tree.
This is the song my tree friend sang to me:

I've got roots growing down to the water,
I've got leaves growing up to the sunshine,
and the fruit that I bear is the sign of life in me.
I am shade from the hot summer sundown.
I am nest for the birds of the heavens.
I'm becoming what the Lord of trees has meant me to be:
A strong young tree.

Trees are a source of beauty either in spring, summer, fall or winter. Yet they can hold many lessons for us as they try to grow tall and strong. Let us pray that we can grow to be trees that the Lord of trees has blessed us to be.

I'm feeling less tired today. It does seem that about one half week after the treatment, my energy level does pick up. I'm finished teaching but I have some important papers to correct yet, so I'm looking forward to having the energy to do that well. I have felt extra pressure in my chest the past few days so I'm going to go in to have my blood pressure taken. It's a side effect that I have to watch. The great news is that the rash on my head is almost cleared up and my feet and hands have lost that tingly feeling and are feeling almost normal once again. In Him.

Wednesday, May 9, 2007 9:01 a.m.

Good Morning,

Last night we attended the preschool graduation of our oldest grandson, Kobi. We as grandparents sat as proud as ever as we watched him sing and recite his line about K being for kindergarten. Besides marveling at how smart he was and how cute he was (that's what grandparents do) we noticed something else. Kobi was the only dark-haired, dark-eyed child on stage. That's because he's half Asian. That gave us cause to marvel too. Not because he's half Asian, but at how his family's journey brought them to northwest Iowa and into our lives.

Souvana's family left Laos, a war-torn country, as refugees in the early 70s. They escaped to Thailand by fleeing through rice paddies at night, giving the young children (including Sou who is the youngest of 14 children) chicken bones to suck on to keep them quiet so as not to alert guards that were in the area. They made it safely to a refugee camp in Thailand where they lived for roughly another nine months before finding a sponsor that would allow them into the United States. There's a lot more to their story but that's it in a nutshell. But what struck me as I watched the graduation was God's providence. How did one family come thousands and thousands of miles, across continents and relocate in our area, allowing a young man to meet our daughter, marry, and provide us with three beautiful grandchildren? All we can say is God's providence. God's providence, the work by which He preserves His world and directs all things to their appointed end:

> The God who made the world and everything in it is the Lord of heaven and earth . . . . From one man he made every nation of men, that they should inhabit the whole earth; and he determined the times set for them and the exact places where they should live. God did this so that men would seek him and perhaps reach out for him and find him, though he is not far from each one of us. "For in him we live and move and have our being." As some of your own poets have said, "We are his offspring." (Acts 17:24a; 26-28)

Through Souvana's family we have seen God's miraculous works. When we reflect on Sou's relocation, we praise God for the work He has done. As I look at my own life, I also see the many ways God's providence is evident. I'm sure you have too. I need to keep trusting that God is sovereign and in control and at the same time He is close and personal. I'm very thankful for His presence in my life. I'm thankful for feeling more energy today. I didn't wake up with a headache this morning, the tingly feeling has left my hands and feet, and the sore in my mouth seems to have healed. Mel, Mindy's friend, took my blood pressure last night and that seems to be staying within an acceptable range. These are all side effects of the medicine. Each day I'm thankful for life and for feeling well enough to enjoy it. I hope you will enjoy this wonderful day that we've been given. In Him.

Thursday, May 10, 2007 9:00 a.m.

Good Morning,

It is a beautiful day in Iowa. The sun is shining and there is a gentle breeze.

My granddaughter Amira is quite a little girl. She provides me with many stories for my college students. Here's a story for you:

Megan went upstairs the other night to tuck Amira in. They have developed a ritual of reading stories and praying. Megan, as she usually does, propped herself on the edge of Amira's bed to pray with her. It was Megan's turn to pray; she prayed that God would take away the rash she was experiencing on her face. Immediately Amira opened her eyes and began to giggle. Megan stopped and asked her what was so funny. Amira, in her very Amira way, smiled up at Megan. Megan knew something was coming. She asked her, "What's so funny?" Amira looked up with a very mischievous look and said, "I'm going to add big spots to the portrait I'm making you for Mother's Day." Megan responded with, "That's not very nice. I don't like these spots. They hurt and they don't look very nice." Even without looking at her, Megan could feel that Amira was just welling up with laughter. She responded, "I know, but I want to do it anyway."

I laughed when Megan told me the story but when I thought about it, I had to admit that there are times in my life that I do the same thing as Amira. Sometimes I know that what I'm going to do is wrong, but the temptation is so great that I choose to disobey. I think of the times I've gossiped, spent my money foolishly or irresponsibly, over ate, and so much more. The desire to sin wells up in me and I make choices to do things I shouldn't. God calls us to be holy. I Peter 1:14-16 says, "As obedient children, do not conform to the evil desires you had when you lived in ignorance. But just as he who called you is holy, so be holy in all you do; for it is written: 'Be holy, because I am holy.'" Our God expects us to imitate Him in all we do and say. He calls us to live a life that glorifies His name. That means turning away from the sinful things that attract us. It's a big assignment, but one we must work at each day and when we do, by the grace of God, we live with a peace that then envelopes our whole being.

By the way, Amira often does make good choices but we are eager to see what Megan's Mother's Day portrait looks like.

I had a very busy day yesterday and it felt good to be able to finish out a day. We are finished with classes but there are still plenty of meetings to attend. Last night after a dinner meeting, I went out with three young women from Dordt who had their hair cut and donated it to me. We went out for smoothies. Another way love has been shown.

Thank you to all of you—for your prayers, for your cards and words of encouragement, for your acts of kindness. Every day I am amazed at who remembers me and how it is done. You are a blessing!

Friday, May 11, 2007 7:31 a.m.

Good Morning,

May is graduation month. On Tuesday we attended the preschool graduation of our grandson. (Kim, I know you had graduation for your students this week too. How did it go?) Soon kindergarten children will walk across the stage and a little later this month so will elementary, middle school, and high school students. Next week our son-in-law, Michael Ribbens, will be graduating from Calvin Seminary. Today the students at Dordt College graduate. That means that many of the students I have worked with for the last four years will be leaving. I'm excited for them to begin the careers that we as an education department have been helping them prepare for and yet there is a feeling of sadness. I will probably never again see some of these students whom I've come to know and love. Sometimes I think about the influence we have over our students. This is especially evident when I read test answers as I did last night. When I read the students' answers, it sometimes scares me. They actually believe what I've said! What a responsibility! I always pray that what I'm telling them is true to God's Word. It is a bit scary sometimes.

It's important for all Christians to remember that no matter what their job, whether they are at work or play, they are always "telling" about what it means to be a Christian. Our daily lives are our test. Sometimes we slip up and the world picks up on that. They see us when we mistreat one another, when we slack off on our work, when we slander, when we lose patience, when we don't live as Christ asks us to. When we talk, others listen. When we act, others watch. As Christians we represent Christ. What a responsibility! God calls us to be salt and light in this world—all the time, everywhere and in every place.

This is the message we have heard from him and declare to you: God is light; in him there is no darkness at all. If we claim to have fellowship with him yet walk in the darkness, we lie and do not live by the truth. But if we walk in the light, as he is in the light, we have fellowship with one another, and the blood of Jesus, His Son, purifies us for all sin. (I John 1:5-7)

I'm feeling great. I even took a two-mile walk last evening. My feet tingled a little afterwards but nothing too bad. It felt good to have the energy to exercise. The fresh warm air felt good too. I'm very thankful for renewed energy. It felt good to put in a full day's work with no nap. I even pulled some weeds yesterday. This is my free week—no chemo yesterday—so I'm hoping I'll be able to keep this energy until my next treatment. I'm looking forward to graduation today and going to Sou's soccer game tonight. I hope you enjoy this beautiful day.

Saturday, May 12, 2007 8:15 a.m.

In the guest book a couple of you mentioned the upcoming holiday that we will celebrate this weekend—Mother's Day. Some of us have mothers with whom we can celebrate and others have the precious memories of their mothers. My mom is a remarkable woman. If you mention her name to many in her community, they will be able to tell you something about her. It might be that they remember her as a caring, capable teacher. Or it might be that they remember her as a choir director. It could be that she sewed their bridesmaid dresses. Maybe they sat beside her at one of her grandchildren's or even great-grandchildren's events. She is a woman of many talents. I'm glad that we have this special day in May to commemorate and celebrate what our mothers mean to us.

My mom has always been very special to me. She has provided me with many wonderful memories. One of my earliest memories is of her reading to us before bedtime. I still have the vivid memory of being banished to the stairsteps as a consequence for something I did (I have no idea what it was). It must have really impacted me though because I still remember the incident clearly. I remember sitting on the bottom step, listening with my ear to the door, trying to catch my mother's voice. I was so jealous of my brother and sister who were each sitting on a side of my mom as she read the story. She was actually very gracious to me, letting me sit on the steps rather than sending me to my room. She knew that I was afraid of being upstairs by myself and so she allowed me to hang out on the steps where I could hear her voice.

Mom provided us with many experiences. She made sure we went swimming in the summer and ice skating in the winter. She took us to the library to get good books and gathered us around the piano to sing with her. When I got older she, along with dad, attended most of my track meets and softball and basketball games, always supporting me whether we won or lost. When I had children she was a wonderful mentor, encouraging and guiding me. She often reminded me to remember that my children were just that—children. She gently told me when I was too harsh and encouraged me when I was too lenient. When I began my teaching career, she was my best teacher. We had many 11:00 p.m. conversations (that's when the telephone rates dropped—true Dutchmen) about curriculum, discipline, and assessment. She taught in various Christian schools for over 45 years. Up until her last day of teaching, she showed me what it was like to be a Christian teacher. She loved her students and wanted what was best for them, just as she did for us, her own children.

But more than anything else, mom has been a wonderful spiritual leader. She taught me how to pray and the importance of reading the Bible. I remember reading the Bible together as a family, each of us having our own Bible so we could be actively engaged. I remember seeing her on her knees praying. She taught us our Bible memory verses and catechism answers. She made sure we were in church every Sunday and I mean every Sunday. (As kids we thought it was unnecessary that she call the county guys to make sure our road was open on Sunday morning.) But she didn't just show us what it meant to have a devotional life; she also showed us how to live the Christian life.

I'm very thankful for my mom. I'm grateful for her guidance, love, and support. I'm also thankful for the heritage that she has passed down. I'm thankful for yet another year that we can celebrate Mother's Day with her. Proverbs 31 describes a woman of strong character, great wisdom, many skills, and a great companion. I'm going to jot down a few but I hope you take the time to read this chapter. I'm sure that like me, you'll find descriptors of your mom too.

> She speaks with wisdom, and
> faithful instruction is on her tongue . . . .
> Her children arise and call her blessed;
> her husband also, and he praises her . . . .
> Charm is deceptive, and beauty is fleeting;
>   but the woman who fears the LORD is to be praised.
> Give her the reward she has earned,
>   and let her works bring her praise at the city gate.
>   Proverbs 31:26, 28, 30, 31

Happy Mother's Day!

I continue to feel good. I'm definitely enjoying the wonderful warm weather. Although yesterday was exhausting, it was a great day. After the graduation ceremony I was able to meet many of my students' parents and congratulate them on their child's success. As I said yesterday, it was sad to say goodbye but it is exciting to see them move on in life. I'm glad for the extra energy although I don't believe it's going to let me get much work finished. I have a shower, reception, and a Dordt party tonight.

Have a great weekend.

Monday, May 14, 2007 8:47 a.m.

In Malachi 3:3 we read: "He will sit as a refiner and purifier of silver . . . ."

The other day Megan sent me the following piece. It gave me much comfort and I thought you might like it too. Some women came across this verse while they were studying the book of Malachi. They were puzzled by it and wondered what this statement meant about the character and nature of God. One of the women offered to find out the process of refining silver and get back to the group at their next Bible Study. That week, the woman called a silversmith and made an appointment to watch him at work. She didn't mention anything about the reason for her interest beyond her curiosity about the process of refining silver. As she watched the silversmith, he held a piece of silver over the fire and let it heat up. He explained that in refining silver, one needed to hold the silver in the middle of the fire where the flames were the hottest as to burn away all the impurities. The woman thought about God holding us in such a hot spot; then she thought again about the verse that says: "He will sit as a refiner and purifier of silver." She asked the silversmith if it was true that he had to sit there in front of the fire the whole time the silver was being refined. The man answered that yes, he not only had to sit there holding the silver, but he had to keep his eyes on the silver the entire time it was in the fire. If the silver was left a moment too long in the flames, it would be destroyed. The woman was silent for a moment. Then she asked the silversmith, "How do you know when the silver is fully refined?" He smiled at her and answered, "Oh, that's easy—when I see my image in it." If today you are feeling the heat of the fire, remember that God has His eye on you and will keep watching you until He sees His image in you. When I'm feeling overwhelmed, distraught, doubting, scared, I need to think about my Refiner and remember that He is watching me—it's good to remember. I hope you do too.

A new week. I continue to feel good, for which I am thankful. I'm hoping the reprieve from treatment last week will bring me into the new series with good counts. I haven't had my blood pressure taken for about a week, but I don't have any indications that it is high. My chest doesn't feel tight nor am I short of breath. My head continues to be free of rash. Yah! My hands and feet are also free from the tingling. Besides feeling tired off and on, I feel close to normal (whatever that is). I'll begin treatments again this Thursday. Please pray that my counts truly are staying in range, and that I can begin this third round strong and healthy. It may sound odd to say, but I'm eager to get started. After this round I can have the PET scan. Thanks for your prayers and other wonderful acts of kindness. Hope your day goes well.

Tuesday, May 15, 2007 10:07 p.m.

Sorry for the late entry today. It was one of those days. I woke up tired but knew that I had to finish my grading so I worked on that until I had to go to a meeting. When I came home I was so exhausted that I went right to sleep. After sleeping away the afternoon, I got up to work on my grading some more. I was hoping not to feel this exhaustion again, but I guess it is going to be part of my life for a while yet.

Tomorrow morning I leave early for the first of the treatments in my third series. It will be a long treatment because I'll get both drugs, the Avastin and Paxil. Although I'm very thankful for the treatments, there certainly are days that I wish I could get rid of all this. I'm trying to make plans for the summer but I'm not sure how much I can actually handle. It's frustrating to plan without knowing if I'll be able to do what I plan. There are many people who have bigger problems than I, so I'm trying to keep that in perspective, but I'd really love to go back to what life was like before January.

While I was writing this, I went to the guest book and I was pleased to see entries from good friends. I checked out the link that Eric suggested and found great encouragement from the sermon that was preached at the evening service at the LaGrave CRC. A passage included in the sermon was Hebrews 12:2: "Let us fix our eyes on Jesus, the author and perfecter of our faith, who for the joy set before him, endured the cross, scorning its shame, and sat down at the right hand of the throne of God." I know the only way I'll get through this exhaustion, the treatments, the unknown future, and everything else is by fixing my eyes on Jesus. I don't have the cross that Christ had to bear, but in a small way I have my own, just as you have your own. When we focus on who God is and the blessings of God, we are reminded that we are not suffering for our sins or our salvation, but through our suffering our faith grows stronger. I pray that the cross you bear makes your faith stronger.

Thursday, May 17, 2007 2:33 a.m.

Good Morning,

As you might guess from my early entry, I am again experiencing energy from the upper that was given with my premeds today. The pattern seems to be quite consistent—after I wake up from the Benadryl, I can't sleep for many hours. After treatment today I had lunch with Vern and Shar (my Sioux Falls relatives), did a little shopping, visited my parents, went to a preschool meeting with Mindy, did the wash, packed our suitcases, answered e-mails, and then finished the last of my grading. Can you see why I love the renewed energy? It may not last for long, but I love it when I have it.

My treatment went well again today. I am thankful for a great team at the cancer center. I'm always treated with respect. The staff was again very pleasant, making my visit enjoyable. Dr. Krie hired a new nurse, someone who had worked in the infusion room so I already knew her. That made that transition easy. My counts were all excellent again today, for which I am very thankful. Even without the Neulasta (the white blood cell booster), my white count is staying right up there. But as I mentioned last week, my blood pressure continues to rise. I was worried for a few minutes during my exam that Dr. Krie was going to hold my treatment, but she decided instead to start me on blood pressure medicine and have me monitor my blood pressure every other day. I asked her if I should get a cuff and try taking it by myself and she said probably not. I guess she knows my nursing talents. This weekend we are going to Michigan to help our son-in-law Michael celebrate his graduation from Calvin Seminary. His parents are going too; his mother is a nurse and agreed to take her cuff along. It will be very handy to have her do this for me and I'm thankful for her willingness to help me. I hope we will see results with the medication.

As I said, we are leaving tomorrow for Michael's graduation. We are proud of him. After four years in college, two years working in Nigeria, and then four years in seminary, he is finally at a milestone for himself. What a great accomplishment! Through all this, he has completed two internships, mentored students in a communal house in a low economic district in Grand Rapids, maintained excellent grades, received a top Calvin Seminary scholarship along with other scholarships, and continued to be a wonderful father and husband. God has blessed him with wonderful gifts and he has chosen to use them for God's glory. I don't say this because he chose to go to seminary, although we are mighty happy with his chosen profession, but because in all he does, we see him as God-honoring and God-fearing.

Life hasn't been easy for Michael and Megan. While their friends were busy establishing themselves in their communities, many getting top-notch jobs and buying nice homes, Michael and Megan have lived as college students (you know what that means). We've never heard them complain about sharing their living space, budgeting for everything, juggling a crazy schedule, and never feeling as if they really belong in a community. They have listened carefully to God's calling and have lived and continue to live their life in tune to His desire for their life.

God calls each of us to be faithful in our lives. That doesn't mean that we will be called to a special ministry but that each one of us, in the jobs we do and in the life that we live, live out our lives for God. God's call for us is to come to Him and be His child. As God calls us to live for Him, we respond by loving Him. Your loving Him has been evident in the way many of you have shown your love to me and I'm sure you have given evidence in many other ways throughout your life. In I Corinthians 1:8, Paul identifies Christians as those who are called "into fellowship with Jesus Christ" (I Thessalonians 2:12). Later he urges Christians to live lives worthy of God, who calls believers into His kingdom.

In following God's call Michael and Megan have chosen to go to Nigeria to work with Nigerian Christians in spreading God's Word. That's their calling. Not all of us are called to that kind of work, but we are all called to do His work, wherever that might be. I'm heading to bed to see if I can get some sleep. Love to all of you.

Friday, May 18, 2007 8:28 a.m.

We made it to Michigan. After my meetings yesterday, Mindy and I took the boys for a quick trip to the Tulip Festival in Orange City. They went on a few rides and then we watched Kim and Ed sing with their bicycle choir. The choir invited the boys to join them for a celebration song which they did with some coaxing from grandma. When Josh finished work and Jerry decided to quit working, we got on the road. I'm always thankful for a safe trip. We're excited for today. Megan has a lot planned for us and tonight we hope to celebrate Mike's great accomplishment by going out to eat.

After all that's happened the past few months, we are thankful for time we can spend with family. We especially treasure these times because we know that all too soon Michael, Megan, Amira, and Nico will be much more than a half-day trip away. But God is good; He's been faithful throughout our life and we know we can count on Him to continue to care for us, just as He cares for you. He has given us many big and little blessings. We're thankful for them all, for the time we can spend with family and friends close to home and far away. I continue to be surprised at all the ways God sends encouragement. When I receive encouragement I often think of the song my young students used to sing: *God Loves a Cheerful Giver.* It's based on II Corinthians 9:6: "Remember this: Whoever sows sparingly will also reap sparingly, and whoever sows generously will also reap generously." That's how I imagine He sees you—as cheerful, generous givers.

So far I'm not feeling any ill effects of the last treatment. The inside of my nose is quite sore but if I keep using the gel that was prescribed for it, it relieves the pain. I'll have my blood pressure taken later today to see what's happening with that. I'm meeting Megan in a few minutes and then who knows what the day will bring. Later.

Friday, May 25, 2007 12:48 a.m.

I'm back. It's been awhile since I've chatted with you. I must have forgotten how to save to the site because I just lost everything I wrote when I went to send my message so I'll try to remember what I wrote.

We had a wonderful time in Michigan. We had a great time with Michael and Megan and the grandkids. Michael's graduation was quite a celebration. We were all very proud of his accomplishment. Even though he did the class work, it truly felt like an accomplishment for the whole family. The ceremony was a celebration of the faithfulness of men and women who followed God's call to a specific task in God's kingdom. We had a great time celebrating with Michael and Megan's friends in the evening. Marilyn (Michael's mom) and I stayed until Tuesday. We both wanted to spend every opportunity we can with Amira and Nico. We had lots of fun swinging, reading books, and playing train.

When I got back on Tuesday night, it was time to think about the week ahead. I had a treatment scheduled for Wednesday morning, but before that I needed to practice with the Sanborn Christian School choir for their graduation in the evening. I couldn't practice with them until 10:30, so I had to make a quick trip to Sioux Falls to try to make my 12:00 appointment. I was nervous on the way down there, wondering if all the excitement in my life the past week would have driven my blood pressure up, and if my counts would allow me to have a treatment. It was great news to hear that everything was okay. My blood pressure had actually dropped, probably a result of the medication I began taking. Dan, the infusion nurse, teased me that maybe, since I was reacting so well, they were just giving me water through my port. That got a rise out of me—he assured me I was really getting chemo, but what a blessing it has been to be able to accept the chemo so well. I am thankful that God allowed my body to accept the treatments.

I have one more treatment in this series (next Wednesday) and then Dr. Krie will set the date for the PET scan. I would like it to be right after the last treatment, but she wants to give that treatment time to work, so it will be either one or two weeks after the treatment. I'm both eager and anxious for the scan. In the meantime we are praying boldly and in faith that God will wipe the spot off my lung. We hold onto His promise to heal, if it be His will. Just as His Word says, He is capable of moving mountains so removing this cancer from me is possible.

I have more I want to share, but it's getting late. I'll write more soon. In Him.

Saturday, May 26, 2007 9:40 a.m.

Good Morning,

As I mentioned earlier in the week, I played for the Sanborn Christian School musical numbers at their graduation ceremony on Wednesday. It was fun to be part of the celebration, watching the faces of the young graduates as they enjoyed every minute of the night and looked with anticipation toward the future. My sister-in-law Karen Bosma was the graduation speaker and she did a wonderful job of explaining the class text from Psalm 40. It is a Psalm of great reassurance that tells us that waiting for God to help us is not always easy, but while we wait, we can serve God. This Psalm (and what Karen said) was for the graduates, but it spoke volumes to me too.

Verses 1-4 say, "I waited patiently for the Lord; he turned to me and heard my cry. He lifted me out of the slimy pit, out of the mud and mire; he set my feet on a rock and gave me a firm place to stand. He put a new song in my mouth, a hymn of praise to our God. Many will see and fear and put their trust in the Lord."

It was the rock that caught my attention. There are times in my life I've tried to set my feet on my own foundation, and it hasn't worked, at least not for long. As I observed the graduation, I realized all the rocks God had put in my life. First of all, he is my rock, the firm foundation that has been revealed to me my whole life. Second, He put many people in my life who were pieces of the rock—my parents, family members, friends, teachers, ministers, neighbors, colleagues, church members, students. Many people have helped me develop a firm place to stand and because of this, I can sing a hymn of praise to God. I must be honest and admit that it is not always easy to sing hymns of praise every minute of the day. There are still times when I sink into the slimy pit, mud, and mire, and at those times I wish to get rid of the medicines, the fatigue, the sores in my mouth, and the pin and needle feeling in my hands and feet. But because of the Rock, those feelings pass and I can put my trust and hope in God. It happens too because of the way the Rock has worked through you. The prayers, the words of encouragement, the acts of kindness are ways that you praise God, but they are also ways that encourage me so that I can praise God. I can never say thank you enough.

The eighth grade class chose a song that meant much to them over the past year; it meant a lot to me too, but in a different way. Here are the words:

> Where do I go when there's no one else to turn to;
> Who do I talk to when no one wants to listen;
> Who do I lean on when there's no foundation stable?
> I go to the Rock I know that's able,
> I go to the Rock.
> I go to the Rock of my salvation,
> Go to the Stone that the builders rejected.
> Run to the Mountain and the Mountain stands by me.
> The earth and all around me is sinking on.
> Where do I hide till the stones pass over;
> Where do I run to when the words of sorrow thunder;
> Is there a refuge in a time of tribulation?
> On Christ the solid Rock I stand
> When I need a shelter
> When I need a friend I go to the Rock.

I'm thankful for the Rock—the one that gives me hope and keeps me strong. I hope all of you are feeling the strength of the Rock in your life too.

By the way Judy, I was just telling someone last night that I have never watched Nemo. Maybe this is a good weekend to pull it out, watch it with Kobi and Bailey, and see what the swimming is about. Except for being tired, I'm feeling great and am looking forward to spending time with family this weekend. Have a good weekend.

Tuesday, May 29, 2007 8:10 p.m.
Hello Everyone,

You'd think with more time on my hands since I'm not teaching, I'd have more time to write on my CaringBridge site. It seems that fatigue has taken care of that. Not only is my body tired but my mind has been tired too. The nurses in the infusion room call it chemo brain. They told me early on that as time went on, it would be more difficult to read and comprehend heavy material and make decisions. That has really proven true. Something else that I've noticed is that stress that I used to take in stride, now wears me out. I played for the church service on Sunday morning and it completely exhausted me. Josh played his trumpet with me during the offertory and since he hadn't done that in a long time, I think I was especially nervous. He did a great job and it was such a joy to play with him once again.

This weekend was a great reminder of the freedoms we have in our country, but on Sunday I was reminded of an even greater freedom that has been given to us, one that we celebrated on Pentecost Sunday—the coming of the Holy Spirit. It was a reminder to me that the presence of God is with us each and every day, helping us live as God wants. This is a huge mystery to me but also a great comfort. I know that I'm not living each day alone; oh, I know, there are many people who are supportive, but even greater than that is a God who walks beside me every day, even when I'm tired and anxious. What a gift! But I must admit, I don't always find it easy to live in the Spirit. Right now I'm experiencing doubt, and as I said, anxiety and fear.

Tomorrow I will have the last of my planned treatments. The last of the three series will be administered. I've looked forward to this day since the beginning of the treatments and yet now that it is here, I'm wondering what's going to happen next. I hope within a week I can have a PET scan which will tell us what is going on in my lung. The big question is: What is happening in my lung? Has the spot shrunk? Could it be possible that it has disappeared? Has it grown? Or has it spread? These are some of the questions that loom in front of me every day. I'm thankful for God's promises, especially His promise that He will never leave me nor forsake me (Joshua 1:5). I know that He will walk with me, no matter what the diagnosis. Please pray that I can rest in His peace the next few weeks as I wait for the results.

Thanks again for all your support and prayers. I was again amazed this weekend at the many people who stopped me and told me they were praying for me. It is truly humbling. In Him.

Thursday, May 31, 2007 12:24 a.m.

Hello my dear friends,

Well, the final administration of the first set of treatments is over. All my counts were good today and my blood pressure was fine so everything went as scheduled. It's kind of crazy to say but treatments are actually quite enjoyable. Dan is the nurse who usually hooks up my drugs. He's great. He has a wonderful sense of humor and his conversations make the time pass quickly. There is always conversation in the infusion room. Each time I take work to do but I never get much finished. Jerry, Josh, Vern and Shar visited with me until I fell asleep and of course, after that, time passes very quickly. The drugs really hit me hard today and I had a difficult time waking up. I was glad Jerry was there to drive me home. I'm feeling fine after the treatment, just fatigued.

Dr. Krie decided to wait three weeks for the PET scan. She knows it will be difficult to wait but since she is going on vacation, there isn't much choice. She could have had me see another doctor for the PET scan report, but we all felt that the wait would be worth it to have her with us when we hear the news. So now the wait begins. It will be long and probably difficult, but I hope that without treatments for about three weeks, I will have energy to work and keep busy. I know I have plenty of work to do. I'm hoping to get a jump start on my course work for next fall. That should keep me plenty busy.

Today was another confirmation of God's grace. He provided me with a knowledgeable and personable doctor and competent nurses, friends, and family who helped the treatment time pass quickly, drugs that can cure, people who keep encouraging me, and prayers from many. I thank Him each day for all that He has done and continues to provide and for the grace that He gives. His grace is amazing and abundant; all we have to do is seek it and we can find it all around us. We all know the message of II Corinthians 12:9: "My grace us sufficient for you, for my power is made perfect in weakness." It holds special meaning for me at this time when I cannot rely on my own power but must rely on God. When I can't rely on my own energy, I know I can count on God to carry me through. The footnote to this text in the NIV Bible essentially says that in our affliction our faith deepens because we admit our weakness and affirm God's strength. I hope that all of you can see God's grace in your life today. It's all around you! Praise God!

One of my favorite songs is "Grace Alone." I'm printing the words, hoping you will enjoy them too.

Ev'ry promise we can make,
Ev'ry prayer and step of faith,
Ev'ry difference we will make
Is only by His grace.
Ev'ry mountain we will climb,
Ev'ry ray of hope we shine,
Ev'ry blessing left behind
Is only by His grace.
Grace alone which God supplies,
Strength unknown he will provide,
Christ in us our Cornerstone;
We will go forth in grace alone.

In Him.

Friday, June 1, 2007 2:23 a.m.

Good Early Morning,

As you might guess from the time of this journal entry, I'm again experiencing unusual sleep patterns. Last night it was extremely late when I finally fell asleep. I actually got much work done before I finally told myself to lie still and hope sleep would come. But tonight is different. I lay down early with Amira and fell asleep, so now I'm finding myself "sleepless in Michigan." Yes, I am in Michigan once again. Jerry surprised me and found a way for me to get here. Eghe is graduating from Grand Rapids Christian High this weekend so I'm hoping to attend her graduation and help Megan with the preparations for her party. It is good to see the whole family once again, but it is especially good to see Amira and Nico. Tonight I met Eghe's family for the first time. It was wonderful to be able to visit with them and learn more about them.

As I said, it is good to see Nico and Amira again. Nico went to bed early but when Amira went to bed, she insisted that we sleep together. Well, that meant reading lots of books first, some books repeatedly, and then singing and telling stories. Tonight she wanted to hear "happy stories" to ward off the bad dreams she was afraid she might have so I told her fun facts about my childhood. I told her about our pony rides, walking by the creek to look for frog eggs, looking at the sky and telling stories by using the pictures we saw in the clouds, going to G'pa and G'ma's house, playing in the haymow, and swinging on the sack swings filled with straw. I'm sure she couldn't comprehend some of the stories because the details were just too old-fashioned for her to picture. As I lay there after she fell asleep, I realized how wonderful my childhood was. I have many happy memories of play times with my brother and sister and my many cousins. I have fond memories of a happy home. I have pleasant memories of family vacations and times just spent on the farm. I don't think I thank God often enough for the heritage I've been given. It is another one of His graces. It was only by God's grace that I was raised in a warm Christian environment.

As I sit here in Michael and Megan's upstairs family room looking out of their front windows, I'm reminded of the twisted environment, the brokenness of shalom that surrounds their house. Just recently they had a drug bust next door and two nights ago a woman who had just been raped came to their house for help. (Nigeria may be safer!) God's creation has surely deviated from His intention. What a responsibility we have, no matter where we live, to try to repair that brokenness.

If you are reading this, you too have probably been blessed by surroundings that were comforting, enriching, and safe. I hope that's the case and if that is so, I hope you too take time to thank God for His abundant grace and gift of love to you.

As I stumbled through the house tonight trying to find things without putting on the lights, I bumped into a chair that I didn't see. I discovered how quickly I can bruise. I decided it probably wouldn't be a good idea for me to get a cut right now. My feet and hands are tingling, but I hope within a day or two this will pass as it has before. I know this is a repeat request, but please continue to pray for not only the drugs to work well, but for me to have peace, the peace that can only come from a wonderful, giving, loving Father. One of God's promises is this: "Peace I leave with you; my peace I give you. I do not give to you as the world gives. Do not let your hearts be troubled and do not be afraid." It's my prayer as I head to bed. In Him.

Tuesday, June 5, 2007 12:58 p.m.

Ah-h-h! Back in Iowa. I had a wonderful time with Megan's family, but it is good to be back home. I slept much when I was there but evidently not quite enough because I slept for a half day when I got home. Fatigue continues to be the battle. It seems I can get myself geared up for what I have to do and then I'm exhausted for a bit of time. One of the best things about being in Grand Rapids was seeing Michael, Megan, and the kids, but it was also wonderful (and astounding) to run into so many people who reminded me that they were praying for me. As I've said a gazillion times, it humbles me, but it also strengthens me. At this point in my life, I know that my healing comes from the Lord. Yes, He has given me a great doctor who prescribed good drugs, but it is God who will heal. And even though I know that God has the power to heal, I sometimes fall into the mindset of, "Will He? Will He choose to heal me?" Hearing from prayer warriors really encourages me.

God does work in mysterious ways. His ways of encouraging me are amazing. For me it was an e-mail from a close friend assuring me that she would pray, even when I couldn't. It was running into Natasha at a graduation party (she is the woman from Michigan who had spots on her lung and is, for now, cancer free) and being able to personally ask her questions and hear her story. It is the constant encouragement I get every single week from one of Jerry's cousins. It even came from a pilot who wished me well.

Another huge encouragement came from two articles that a friend sent from the book *God's Two Minute Warning* by John Hagee. The first article gave many biblical references to the many ways God has miraculously worked throughout biblical history. He miraculously made the world; He divided the Red Sea; He saved the three men in the fiery furnace. The Son also had a ministry based on miracles. He healed the blind, the lame and the lepers. He raised a dead boy and a man from his grave. Miracles happen differently today, but they do happen. Check out James 5. In his book James called on the church to keep praying and believing in miracles.

The devotional gave some good advice on where to find miracles. He said, "You can find miracles in cans! When you start saying, 'I can do all things through Christ who strengthens me,' you are fostering a miracle mentality. Begin to say, 'I can have a better marriage,' 'I can be free from the chains of alcohol and drug addiction,' 'I can be healed from this dreaded disease in my body,' 'I can climb this impossible mountain.'"

One of the stumbling blocks the devotional suggested was fear, and it is one that lives in my life if I let it. Scripture says, "For God has not given us a spirit of fear, but of power and of love and of a sound mind" (II Timothy 1:7, NKJV). Jesus often told his disciples "Fear not." He reminds us not to fear poverty, illness, the past, and even death.

The author also reminded his readers of another stumbling block— doubt. God continuously reminds believers to have faith in Him. "Doubt is like a cancer that destroys your faith in God. Rather than entertaining your doubts, feed your faith." Doubt can be a major obstacle in our spiritual progress. Having faith in God can lead to the impossible. I'm praying for a miracle and the faith to hold on until I hear the good news. Thanks for your prayers and other ways you encourage. I hope you too, if you have doubts in your life, are holding on to the lifeline that comes from God.

Tuesday, June 5, 2007 10:50 p.m.
Hello friends,

A book called *Humankind* graces the top of the coffee table in Mike and Megan's living room. Megan loves photography and has purchased some wonderful books on the subject but I believe this is the best book in her photography library. Yoshio and Eiko Komatfu have taken photographs around the world for 35 years. They've taken their collection and put photos under themes like love, hope, hurt, belief, play, rest, and need. One them I found very interesting. Along with pictures of people doing a variety of activities was the quote, "By the work one knows the workman"—Jean de La Fontaine. Isn't that a great quote?

This quote can be interpreted in many ways but I chose to look at it as it relates to my Christian life. By my work, others know who I am, who I am aligned to. Lately I've been reading books to help me write devotions for the mission team from our church that is going to Cary, Mississippi. Many of the books emphasized the importance of showing love to those on the team and to those who are being ministered to. By our actions we show who Christ is. When we speak kindly, when we show kindness to others, when we respect others, when we are patient, when we are joyful, among other things, we show who Christ is. That doesn't mean we have to give up our convictions, but that we show our convictions in a loving way. I'm not sure when we decided that harshness and beating people over the head was a good way to spread the gospel. In Galatians 5:22 & 23a we read: "But the fruit of the Spirit is love, joy, peace, patience, kindness, goodness, faithfulness, gentleness, and self-control." These fruits don't just show up in us—the Spirit grows these fruits in us as we strive to imitate Christ. Our work is to be more like Christ. When we do this, we fulfill the intended purpose of the law—to love God and our neighbor. Have a good day spreading God's love!

Thursday, June 7, 2007 12:25 a.m.
Hello dear friends,

It has been another fatiguing day. It seems each morning I just can't wake up. I finally felt awake enough to get out of the house this afternoon. I went to visit my parents. Mom and I did a little shopping for some new accessory pieces for her living room. It was good to get out for awhile. I'm hoping that as I get further and further away from my last treatment, my energy level will pick up. My mouth sores and the tingling in my feet and hands have improved greatly over the last twenty-four hours. I'm very thankful for that.

Each day I mentally count off the days to my PET scan. I wish I wasn't so obsessed by the scan but I must admit that it does consume much of my thinking. This is probably adding to my fatigue. I have such mixed feelings running through me. I don't want to set myself up for disappointment but I also want to believe that I can be healed. For days I've been struggling with this and then tonight I came across Psalm 112:7. In the Living Bible it reads, "He does not fear bad news, nor live in dread of what may happen. For he is settled in his mind that Jehovah will take care of him." The last part of that verse is the key. It all boils down to my trust in my Creator. I'm afraid that sometimes I'm only seeing God as a God who cares for me if I'm healed. I have to believe and have faith that God will care for me even if my lung isn't healed. Even if the spots remain, I have to trust that God will carry me through that too. God's perfect love is too difficult to comprehend in a world where love is often conditional and temporary. The truth is God is able to keep me secure in His perfect plan even when my fears threaten to sweep over me. He will keep me secure even if I don't hear that my lung is cancer free.

I praise you God for who You are. In your word You say that You will never leave me or forsake me. Your love is never-ending. You have always been faithful and I know that I can count on your faithfulness to continue. I am grateful that I can cast all my cares on You (Psalm 55:22), not because of who I am but because of who you are. I praise you for your perfect love.

Friday, June 8, 2007 2:49 p.m.

Good Day,

The wind has been awful. Those gale gusts have been enough to make one tired. My own beautiful plants have taken a beating but they seem to have weathered the storm well enough to continue showing off their beauty. When I looked out this morning, I saw a much gentler breeze brushing against the tree leaves. I hope it stays that way.

This was another great lesson on life for me. I've felt many stormy days the past week. I continue to battle fatigue and soreness and added with that, the insecurity of doubt and fear. It doesn't take much for me to fall into a tearful mood. And then I thought about what I was observing in nature. Isn't it something how God uses nature to reveal Himself to us? Those stormy, windy days have passed; oh, they may return, but before they come again, God has sent a reprieve. A time for our plants to strengthen, a time for them to be nourished, and a time for them to develop deeper roots. This doesn't happen instantly but with time. Every time a storm comes and the plants survive, they become stronger. All this so that their beauty can give us joy, inspire us, and relax us.

I've felt worn out the past two days—wind-blown and hanging on. But I know, because I know who holds my future, calm days will follow. The wind will stop and so will the anxiety. Beauty will once again be restored as I receive spiritual nourishment and my roots deepen. The storms will come again, I can be sure of that, but I also have the surety that next time I will be stronger. If you are going through a storm in your life, hang on, fight hard, and don't let go. Better times are coming but don't just wait for them—search the scriptures, pray, seek out good friends, walk close to God.

In Ephesians 3:14-19 we read: "For this reason I kneel before the Father, from whom his whole family in heaven and on earth derives its name. I pray that out of his glorious riches he may strengthen you with power through his Spirit in your inner being, so that Christ may dwell in your hearts through faith. And I pray that you, being rooted and established in love, may have power, together with all the saints, to grasp how wide and long and high and deep is the love of Christ, and to know this love that surpasses knowledge—that you may be filled to the measure of all the fullness of God."

Thanks for praying that my roots may grow deeper and through that I can shine forth with the beauty of Jesus Christ. In Him.

Monday, June 11, 2007 1:02 a.m.

Yesterday was a difficult day. During the morning church service we had the commissioning service for the Cary, Mississippi SERVE Project. The SERVE team will be leaving this week for Cary and Glen Allen. I've been a part of this mission outreach for eleven years and Jerry has gone with the team for six years. It is difficult to think about not going with the team. It's not that I think they can't get along without us; they have very capable leaders and team members but both of us are going to miss the joy we've experienced over the past years by being a part of this team. As is said of most short-term mission trips, people who go to witness probably receive more than they give. We hope that in some way God has used us over the past years to make a difference in lives, but we know that we have been tremendously blessed by the people we have worked with at the Cary Christian Center and Straight Gate Ministry. Both of these organizations have taught us what it really means to be a servant. They've 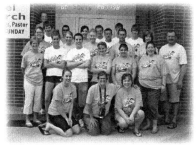 shown us what it means to live a life of giving. They've also taught us much about other cultures and how to respond to them. Our lives have also been enriched and blessed by the children we've come to know. Both of us will miss their smiling faces, warm hugs, and entertaining conversations. We will miss sharing God's Word with them. But we realize that this year it isn't meant to be. God has other plans for us this summer. Even though I've shed many tears about not going and will miss the opportunity to connect with my Mississippi friends, I'm thankful that there are people who've been willing to pick up the work and make it possible for the project to continue.

This summer we won't be witnessing in Mississippi; that's hard, but it has reminded me that I need to be conscious of witnessing for Him around my community. There are many opportunities that I can take advantage of if only I look around. I'm praying God will give me the energy and open my eyes to opportunities close to home. When Megan was home last time, she reminded me to think about doing one thing each week to encourage or help someone. I believe that is my assignment for this summer. There are widows I've neglected; there are sick whom I haven't taken time for and so many other ways that I can serve.

God asks us to be His witnesses in His world; it doesn't have to be in a far-away place. Actually I've found it easier to witness to the strangers I've met in Mississippi than to my neighbors back home. I love what I Peter 3:15 says: "But in your hearts set apart Christ as Lord. Always be prepared to give an answer to everyone who asks you to give the reason for the hope that you have. But do this with gentleness and respect . . . ." I hope I can witness even here in my neighborhood this summer to a Savior who's given His life for me. I hope you can too.

In Him.

Tuesday, June 12, 2007 12:31 a.m.

Hello dear friends,

Last week I had coffee with a couple of old friends. Marlys Vander

Pol, who now lives in Washington, has been a friend since grade school. We spent much time ice skating, playing ball, talking about boys, and hanging out when we were young. Starla Reitsma has been a friend since high school; our children grew up together and we share activities in church. We had a great time laughing and reminiscing about old times. Mar reminded me of the time we were walking from the campus commons at Dordt to our dorm. The wind, like the wind last week, was horrendous. It was so strong, in fact, that we formed a line and hung onto each other as we made our way back to the dorm. I was at the end of the line and somehow my hold on the next person broke. Immediately I was torn from the group, picked up by the wind; it threw me on the hood of a parked car. It must have been quite a sight! We did agree that this probably wouldn't happen today. (If you don't get why, just check the weight difference.) This experience taught us the importance of sticking together. The strength of a group is obvious in many situations. Soccer players stand in a close line to protect the goal when there is a penalty kick. When children play Red Rover, they form a line and they hold tightly to one another to keep their line from breaking. Often inexperienced singers find strength in standing close by singers who are singing their part. It's true in life! When we stick together, we accomplish more. Ecclesiastes 4:9-12 says: "Two are better than one, because they have a good return for their work: If one falls down, his friend can help him up. But pity a man who falls and has no one to help him up! Also, if two lie down together, they will keep warm. But how can one keep warm alone? Though one may be overpowered, two can defend themselves. A cord of three strands is not quickly broken."

God designed life for companionship, not isolation. He doesn't expect us to live for ourselves but to serve God and others. He encourages us to be team members. I have been wonderfully blessed by others and I thank God for that. All through life, others have shown me compassion, love, and companionship. It has been the thing that has carried me through many stressful situations. Right now I couldn't stand to be going it alone. Tonight I went for a walk by myself and by the time I got home I had fabricated all kinds of scary scenarios for the future. But when I got home I was lifted up by the companionship of friends through cards, phone calls, e-mails and CaringBridge journals. Arlene, my sister-in-law, stopped over to take my blood pressure and we had an uplifting conversation. "If one falls down, his friends can pick him up." I continue to feel the effect of this verse. I'm thankful for the companionship of friends and family.

My blood pressure had been going up and down but tonight it was down. I'm thankful for that. Today I reaped the effects of a busy weekend and even though I was able to get some work done this morning, this afternoon was a wash-out. I ended up trying to sleep off a headache most of the afternoon. Jerry was happy to have me help him with the watering this evening. It helped cut his watering time in half and it felt good for me to be outside getting some fresh air. I keep discovering new sores in my mouth, am struggling with headaches, and am retaining much fluid in my hands, so I think I'll call the clinic tomorrow and see if they have any ideas on what I can do for these issues. Thanks for your prayers and other acts of kindness. In Him.

Wednesday, June 13, 2007 9:49 a.m.

Hello dear friends,

Talk about grace. Yesterday I experienced the epitome of grace. Here's what happened: Before I was diagnosed with cancer, I had registered for two graduate courses at University of South Dakota. As those of you who are close to me know, I didn't have a very realistic picture of what my life was going to be like for the next six months. In fact, after I was diagnosed, I attended a meeting with my department and told them I'd probably be out a few days, but if they could help cover those days, I would be back to my regular teaching schedule. Well, that didn't exactly happen. I was out of the classroom for the first half of the semester and then came back with only half my classes the last part. I'll be forever grateful for my colleagues' foresight when I had none. I didn't drop my on-line courses, one reason being the drop/add period had elapsed by the time I realized what I was in for. So, being a little unrealistic, well, maybe a lot unrealistic, I stayed in the classes. To make a long story short, I kept up quite well with one of the courses until the very end and I failed miserably to complete the work in the other. Yesterday I made the trip to USD to see if there was any way I could salvage the semester. I had many emotions that made that trip with me. I was angry at myself for not finishing; I was embarrassed by my lack of performance; I felt humiliated and all kinds of other negative feelings. I've been praying hard the past few weeks for the courage to make the plunge and talk to the professors and yesterday was the day. It didn't take me long after I walked into the education building at USD to feel the love and compassion of the instructors. They assured me that they would allow me to finish my uncompleted work and on my time. They were willing to adjust the courses to meet my needs. I was overwhelmed with gratitude at the grace they showed to me. I was amazed that they would do this for me. They didn't have to, but they did.

Isn't that like God's amazing grace? He didn't have to send His Son to die for us, but He chose to because He loves us. Every day we are recipients of His love, even if we don't take notice of it. I used to think grace was giving me what I thought I wanted—making me better, providing a problem-free life. But after experiencing some trials in my life, I now know that His grace is much more. His grace means that He can heal me, but His grace might be helping me through a traumatic situation, holding me close as I grieve or struggle or mourn. Yesterday His grace was shown through two wonderful women and I thank Him for this wonderful gift.

I've referred to this verse before but yesterday it came to life for me again. Paul says in II Corinthians 12:8-9: "Three times I pleaded for the Lord to take it away from me. But he said to me, 'My grace is sufficient for you, for my power is made perfect in weakness.' Therefore I will boast all the more gladly about my weaknesses, so that Christ's power may rest on me." Each day I thank God for His grace, His grace that shows up through all of you. In Him.

Wednesday, June 13, 2007 10:36 p.m.

My dear friends,

Paul wrote the book of Philippians for the church in Philippi. He wanted to thank the believers for helping him when he had a need. Even though he was imprisoned, he wanted the people to know that he was full of joy. Philippians 1:3 says: "I thank God every time I remember you." I'm not Paul, but I think I have an inkling of what he was feeling. You know that lately I've been feeling the burden of not knowing what the future holds for me but God has sent many of you to bring me joy. Today my friend Pat came and helped me finish up my gardens. I just couldn't make up my mind how to fill in the empty spaces and she not only helped me pick out flowers, she also dug the holes! I received a wonderful CD, a luminary bag from a friend in Fulton, Ilinois, and more encouraging cards, e-mails, phone calls, and journal entries. You have brought me much joy.

The footnote in my Bible says that by helping Paul, the Philippians were helping Christ's cause. "The Philippians were willing to be used by God for whatever He wanted them to do. When others think about you, what comes to their minds? Are you remembered with joy by them? Do your acts of kindness lift up others?" I am remembering you with joy.

Your acts of kindness are definitely lifting me up. Thank You! Just a little note: I stayed awake all day today! That may sound funny to you, but that's a first in many days for me. Not only did I stay awake but I kept busy all day. It was a great feeling. Maybe I'm over the hump of constant fatigue. I hope so.

Friday, June 15, 2007 9:19 a.m.

Good Morning,

Neither Jerry nor I handled the Cary SERVE team send-off very well today. I wanted to be strong; I didn't want to draw attention to myself, but it was too difficult. When they got in their vehicles and closed the doors, the tears came. It just didn't seem right. But later in the day, I already knew it was right that I didn't go. I don't know if it was the emotionalism from the morning or just the fatigue from chemo, but I slept for the entire afternoon. This fatigue is different from the tiredness I've experienced before. When it hits me, I have no choice but to rest. The fatigue usually begins and ends with a severe headache. When I wake up it feels as if I've just struggled to climb out of a long tunnel. So even though it was hard to see the team leave without us, I know it was the best decision. Kobi and Bailey are planning to stay overnight on Saturday night and Mike and Megan are coming home toward the beginning of next week so we have much to look forward to. And of course, the PET scan and diagnosis will come next week.

My cries to God have increased. I wish that I didn't have to admit that adversity brings me closer to God, but that is exactly what has happened. I always hope that my line of communication stays strong when I'm healthy and trouble free, but I know that isn't true. When I read Psalm 86, I see that the same thing happened to David. In his troubled times he too sought God most intensely. I hope you take time to read the whole Psalm but here are some verses that mean much to me:

> Hear, O Lord, and answer me,
> for I am poor and needy.
> Guard my life, for I am devoted to you.
> You are my God; save your servant,
> who trusts in you.
> Have mercy on me, O Lord,
> for I call to you all day long.
> Bring joy to your servant,
> for to you, O Lord,
> I lift up my soul . . . .

Teach me Your way, O Lord,
and I will walk in your truth;
give me an undivided heart,
that I may fear your name.
I will praise you, O Lord my God, with all my heart!
I will glorify your name forever.
For great is your love toward me;
you have delivered me from the depths of the grave.

What a beautiful Psalm. I hope you will take time to read all of it. God is a gracious and compassionate God, and I especially see this when I face trials. Have a good day. Look for God's goodness. In Him.

Saturday, June 16, 2007 11:00 a.m.

I'm sitting here this morning working on one of my USD classes and I'm bouncing in my chair as I'm typing. Yes, I do feel energized this morning even after an exhausting night last night (but more about that later). Earlier this morning someone asked me if I was missing Cary and guess what—I immediately had tears in my eyes. So I decided if I can't be there, I can get a little piece of it. I found one of the Cary music CDs and began to listen to the songs that we have sung over the years—songs that bring strong memories of the children and the people we love dearly down there. (It even includes "Precious Lord," Ed.) I'm not down there in person, but I am going to do my best to experience what I can right here in Sanborn. Along with the upbeat and spirited music, I walked outside to enjoy the wonderful warm and humid weather. That's a part of the Cary experience too. That may seem a little crazy to you, but I love it. Besides keeping up with the website, Jerry or I talk to the team a couple of times a day so we feel as if we are on a virtual trip with them.

Sometimes things don't go as we plan or even how we would like them to go; that's when a flexible and positive attitude becomes helpful. I always tell student teachers I supervise that there are good lessons to be learned from a negative student-teaching placement and that's how it is in life too. When plans get changed, when we don't have control over what happens, when we don't like what we are experiencing, it is important to look for the good or the lessons that can be gleaned from the experience. Even things we might see as negative in our life can help us grow. I can already see growth happening in me. Again I'm seeing how God gently provides for us.

Last night we participated in the O'Brien cancer survivor and memory walk. It was a very touching and memorable experience. The evening began with a survivor's walk. I joined them. I don't know what God has in store for me, but I'm surviving right now and I'm feeling excited about life. We probably walked between three and four miles with friends, acquaintances, and those we didn't know. When dusk came, they lit the luminary bags; it was a breathtaking experience. I don't know God's plan for me but I do know that right now He is holding me in the palm of His hand and He's not only making me comfortable, He's also providing me with a life that is full and exciting. Again, I thank God for this. I like the message God gives in Jeremiah 17:7-8: "But blessed is the man who trusts in the LORD, whose confidence is in him. He will be like a tree planted by the water that sends out its roots by the stream. It does not fear when heat comes; the leaves are always green. It has no worries in a year of drought and never fails to bear fruit." Oh, to be like that tree!

You've again blessed me with your inspirational CaringBridge journal entries. Your words have lifted me up, made me laugh and cry, and shown me a piece of who God is: loving, caring, kind, encouraging, understanding, just to name a few characteristics.

Just for your information—I'm listening to a song that the Glen Allen kids love to sing. It's called "Never Give Up." It tells us that we are never to give up because God is always there; He is always by our side, at any time and anywhere. What a reminder!

By the way, Mar Sjaarda, thanks for the pink ribbon socks. They really made my feet comfortable on the walk. I looked pretty snazzy in my pink-ribboned socks and the pink-ribboned Twins hat that Josh gave me!

Love you all! I hope you find God's blessing in your day too.

Monday, June 18, 2007 12:54 a.m.

We spent the weekend celebrating Father's Day. On Saturday night we went to the park with my extended family. It was wonderful to see four generations celebrating together. I can't imagine the feeling my dad must have had as he watched his youngest great-grandchild toddling through the grass, to having conversations with his children. What a blessing to see God's faithfulness throughout the generations. Many of us attend different churches, but we all honor and serve the same God. And to think that all of this is happening because we had a father who was faithful to God and listened to His call to raise up his children in a godly way. That doesn't mean that our family doesn't have problems and that we haven't made mistakes. We have made and will continue to make mistakes, but because of the faithfulness of our parents, we have had instruction and modeling on how to live as Christians. Integrity, honesty, compassion, patience, and being servants are some of the qualities we witnessed as we grew from children to adulthood. I'm thankful for the blessing and the gift of a father who loved and continues to love God.

The count-down is beginning. There is only one day left before the PET scan and then one more day before we hear the results. I'm amazed at how God has calmed my heart. I'm thankful for all the prayers that have been said on my behalf. I won't say that I still don't experience some anxious moments but generally I'm feeling assurance that God will walk especially close to me these next few days. He has provided me with many encouraging words through scripture, devotionals, and words from people. Tonight I read about William Cooper. During a very bleak time in his life he tried to take his life. He swallowed poison, but it failed. He hired a driver to take him to the Thames River where he intended to hurl himself over the bridge but was somehow restrained. The next day he fell on a sharp knife but the blade broke. He then tried to hang himself but was found in time to save his life. Shortly after these failed attempts on his life, he read the book of Romans where he met the God of storms and found peace. Sometime later he wrote these familiar words: "God moves in a mysterious way His wonders to perform; He plants His footsteps in the sea, and rides upon the storm. Deep in unfathomable mines of never-failing skill He treasures up His bright designs, and works His sovereign will."

Life is filled with storms. Each of us has our own storms. Your storm is different than mine. Yet all of us can be assured that God is in control of these storms. I'm not sure how His sovereign will is going to be worked out through my storm, but I do know that through it, God has shown Himself to me in powerful ways. In many ways He has assured me that He is walking beside me. This experience has brought me to my knees to look to Him for my strength.

In Romans 8:28 we read: "And we know that in all things God works for the good of those who love him." I don't know what that good is going to look like, but I know it will fulfill His purpose. Please continue to pray for us as we face these next few days. Thank you!

Tuesday, June 19, 2007 1:16 a.m.

Dear friends,

As I contemplate what will happen over the next few days, I wish I could fast-forward to Wednesday around noon. By that time the PET scan would be over and the diagnosis would be told. But that isn't possible so the next best thing, or maybe the best thing, is to remember that my life is in the hands of God, just as yours is. Whatever happens, good news or bad, God will be by my side. I know I can count on many of you being by my side too, maybe not literally but in spirit and in prayer.

Tomorrow I will have a dye injected into my port around 12:30. Then I will have to lie perfectly quiet in a dark room for about 45 minutes before they scan me. The whole process should take about two hours. I'm thankful for the port; I'm thankful for wonderful technicians; I'm thankful for modern medicine and sophisticated machines; I'm thankful for a couple of good movies (at least relatively good) that are on tonight so that I can have my time occupied until I'm tired enough to fall asleep; I'm thankful for a skilled and caring doctor; I'm thankful for compassionate infusion nurses; I'm thankful for my family and friends who have supported me and continue to support me through this journey; I'm thankful for prayer; I'm thankful to Christ who gives new life; I'm thankful for the Spirit who continues to work in my life and in yours; and I'm thankful to God for the peace He has given me.

A verse familiar to all of you is one that I am concentrating on tonight: "Trust in the Lord with all your heart and lean not on your own understanding; in all your ways acknowledge him and he will make your paths straight" (Proverbs 3:5-6).

Again, thanks for all the ways you have shown Christ to us.

Jerry and Cella

Tuesday, June 19, 2007 11:17 p.m.

Good Evening,

I'm so exhausted that I hardly have the energy to type this message, but I wanted all of you to know. Today I had the PET scan and it was pretty routine. I slept through much of it so time passed quickly. When I was ready to leave I asked the technicians, who, by the way, were as gracious as last time, if the results would get to Dr. Krie by tomorrow morning. They didn't think their delivery service would be able to get the scan delivered by 9:00 so I volunteered to deliver the package. As I got in the car with the scan, you don't know how much I wanted to peek at the scan. But I knew it wouldn't be a good idea. After we dropped it off, Megan and I went to Hobby Lobby to do a little shopping. While I was there my phone rang, and as one always does, I glanced at the caller ID and saw Dr. Krie's name. It had been such a short time since we had dropped the scan off that I couldn't imagine that she had read the scan already, but she had. The first thing she said was, "Cella, the spot that we biopsied is gone. It's really gone." I couldn't believe what I was hearing. It was such a shock! I didn't know what to do. First of all I found Megan and told her. The people in the store must have thought we had lost it. The next thing I did was call Jerry, Mindy, and Joshua. They, of course, were completely shocked that I had already heard the results and were totally overjoyed! Pam Adams, one of my colleagues, was also in the store, so we excitedly shared the news with her too.

I'm still in shock. I've been waiting for this news for a long time. I expected to have to wait one more night, but the wait is over. I can't begin to tell you my feelings. I'm just exhausted from all the emotions. When Dr. Krie told me the news all I could say was, "Praise God!" That was the response of many that I talked to today. What else can we say? God has been good. He's always good and even if the news would have been less positive, we know God would have been good but we really experienced His grace and love today.

Tonight my heart is singing—so many songs and texts are running through my head, but the song that tops them all is a song we sing when we arrive in Cary:

"Praise God from whom all blessings flow. Praise him all creatures here below. Praise him above ye heavenly host, Praise Father, Son and Holy Ghost."

Thank you, God! Thank you, CaringBridge readers, for all your prayers. Thank you for your support. Please join us in thanking and praising God for His immeasurable care.

I'll post more tomorrow about the treatments that are to come. Although the largest spot is gone there is still one nodule on the lung, so Dr. Krie wants me to begin a new series already tomorrow. I need to be on the road by 7:00 so that means I've got to try to get some sleep.

In Him, Jerry and Cella

Thursday, June 21, 2007 8:07 a.m.

Dear friends,

Last evening (after I finally woke up after my treatment) I went outside to water our flower gardens. We have gardens that circle our house. Each year we add to the gardens so we have some established flowers and some that have recently been added. Both of us have taken on different jobs in our gardens. Jerry's jobs include digging holes for new plants, landscaping around the gardens, and watering. He weeds if I'm standing close and can tell him which "green things" are plants and which are weeds. I pick out most of the plants, weed, dead-head, and occasionally water. When I walked outside I noticed that some of our flowers were looking a little droopy. We haven't gotten any of the area showers lately so the ground is a little water deprived. Most of our drooping flowers were planted very recently. They still haven't established a root system. I decided that it would be better for the newly planted flowers if I popped off the flowers so that the energy could go to establish the plant. It pains me to pop off those beautiful blooms. The vivid colors, the size, shape, and height of the plant are the reason I chose the plant. I don't usually consider the leaves when I'm shopping for new plants. But I also know that if energy can go to establish the plant, soon the beautiful flowers will pop up from a flourishing plant. (See, Donna, I've learned a few things from you!)

Unfortunately, I don't always feel like a rooted plant. I still fall into doubt and fear and discontent. Tuesday I was ecstatic after I heard the results of my PET scan. And yet one day later after talking with Dr. Krie, I fell into the category of a new plant. I was still thrilled that the spots were gone, but I was disconcerted by the great possibility they will come back. The spots may come back if I have to stop the drug treatment I am on because of reactions or because it is no longer effective. Once this happens, Dr. Krie will change drugs to see if another drug will be effective and there is a great possibility it will be, but I wonder. And that means constant chemo. It's hard for me to think about that. When I asked her how many of her patients have beaten the disease, she said she could think of one patient who has made it ten years and that is pretty much in line with what other doctors report. I was devastated at the statistics but then I had to remind myself that I am not a statistic; I am a child of God and He will determine what will happen to the cancer in my body.

I remember what Corrie Ten Boom once said after suffering in a German concentration camp during WW II: "When the train goes through a dark tunnel and the world gets dark, do you jump off? Of course not. You sit still and trust the engineer to get you through." So I'll cling to God, praying He will engineer me through any tunnel that comes my way.

"But the LORD still waits for you to come to him so he can show you his love and compassion. For the LORD is a faithful God" (Isaiah 30:18 NLT).

Thanks for all your words of encouragement. Your prayers hold me tight and lift me up. In Him.

Saturday, June 23, 2007 9:32 a.m.

Hi,

A quick note to say that I attended a conference on diverse learning the past few days. I'm hoping to head out to my brother's farm to take the kids horseback riding. Doesn't that sound like fun? I'll post more later. Have a wonderful day!

Monday, June 25, 2007 12:55 a.m.

Dear friends,

I imagine if you read my last journal entry, you probably recognized a small sense of fear. I wanted badly to relish in the great news of the disappearance of the cancer and yet when I heard Dr. Krie talk about the future, fear and uncertainty crept in. Realistically, I'm afraid of constant chemo. I'm afraid when I think of the fatigue I feel and my teaching schedule this fall. I wonder how long I'll really be able to stay on this effective treatment that is controlling the cancer. I wonder if another treatment will work if I have to change chemos. All these questions and no answers. In my humanness, I want answers and I'd like them loud and clear. I know God is capable; I know He can be loud and clear, but more often than this response, we hear God in gentle whispers, gentle whispers that come as hugs, words of encouragement, quiet stories from faithful people, words of truth from the Bible. I need to keep my eyes and ears open to the gentle whispers of comfort, peace, and assurance. When I feel the roller coaster jolting for a ride, I realize that I don't need to hang on as much as I need to wait patiently and be still and remember who God is. I need to remember God's promises and His faithfulness. If I remember these things, I will receive grace in the right portion, grace that will sustain me in my present need.

I Kings 19:11-12 reads: "The LORD said, 'Go out and stand on the mountain in the presence of the LORD . . . .' Then a great and powerful wind tore the mountains apart . . . but the LORD was not in the wind . . . there was an earthquake, but the LORD was not in the earthquake . . . fire, but the LORD was not in the fire. And after the fire came a gentle whisper."

Wednesday, June 27, 2007 7:29 a.m.

Good Morning,

I love to watch my grandchildren. I've really been full of joy the past few weeks because I was able to enjoy all five of my grandchildren. Their energy, love for life, and trust amaze me. I watched them as they ran on the track and in between the track, and off the track at the Relay for Life last Friday night. Nothing could stop them. As they ran, dodged and jumped, they giggled and laughed and were as silly as could be. They also showed trust as they took off around the track, leaving us "in the dust" assuming we would still be there when they finished their run. They trusted that their little legs would bring them around the track to the spot where they began. Not so with us—once we started around that first bend, we hoped we would make it back to the finish line. What a lesson that evening was for me. It reminded me once again that I have to trust that God will bring me full circle, that He will bring me around the track. The best way I can hold on to that trust is by once again becoming like a little child. I need to have the faith that a child has, a faith that says I can trust God. So often my trust or distrust relies on my experiences, on what I know, on what I've seen, on what I read on the Internet, and yet God says we are to put our trust in Him—like a child. What should appear so easy, so simple, is difficult for me. I struggle with trying to pave my own way. I rely on myself to get through life and yet God says that whoever comes to Him as a little child will have eternal life.

David says in Psalm 8: "O LORD, our LORD, how majestic is your name in all the earth! You have set your glory above the heavens. From the lips of children and infants you have ordained praise." Children are able to trust and praise God without doubts or reservations. As we get older, sometimes we find this more difficult. I need to give God my child-like faith, removing any barriers that make it difficult for me to trust Him.

My sleep patterns are again out of kilter. Last Wednesday and Thursday nights were almost sleepless. Sleepless in Sanborn! I wonder if I could write a movie script on this? Then came along a busy Saturday and Sunday. (We got to hear Michael preach and present in two different churches on Sunday. We are thrilled with Mike and Megan's conviction and passion for the work they will soon begin.)

That meant that on Monday and Tuesday I was extremely fatigued. Jerry says I should try to cut out most things, but I only have Amira and Nico here for a few more days, so I'm willing to be tired in order to spend time with them. Monday I went swimming with all the grandkids. It was great. (The kids even thought my new swimming cap was pretty cool.) Although Nico and Miles slept most of the time, Kobi, Bailey, and Amira loved swimming with me in the big pool. I did come home exhausted (meaning I slept from 4 p.m. until 8 a.m.), but it was worth it. When I fall into these fatigue modes, I have no energy. Nilcho! It's a weird phenomena for me and one I don't like very much. I want badly to get up and begin checking off those things I have on my list, but here's where again, I have to put my trust in God. I have to believe that even if I don't accomplish all I have planned, things will be okay. Have a good day.

Thursday, June 28, 2007 8:44 a.m.

Good Morning,

I was hoping to write more in my journal this morning, but between the fatigue and finishing up an on-line course, I just haven't had time. I'm leaving in a few minutes for my second treatment in this new set of treatments. I'm hoping it goes as well as the past treatments. Actually, I'll probably be up the next two nights so I'll write then. Have a good day.

Friday, June 29, 2007 8:53 a.m.

Dear friends,

God is so good! He has been working in my heart. Even with the good news I got last week, I must admit that my heart has been unsettled. Let me explain. Isn't it funny how joys in your life can actually work against you? It has been wonderful to have our whole family together the last few weeks, doing so many fun things together. But at times it seemed bittersweet. We spent a lot of time laughing, relaxing, talking, all the kinds of things you do with those you love. But sometimes I would sit back and wonder, "How long? How many more times?" I loved watching Kobi jump off the diving board and Bailey and Amira get more used to the water. I just giggled when I saw Nico's great big smile when it was announced that we were leaving the pool (he doesn't like the water). And it was calming to watch Miles sleep through the whole experience. But through it all, plus so many encouraging comments from so many of you, God has worked peace in my heart.

There's a song titled "He Knows How to Care for What Belongs to Him." When I sang the words to this song, I once again realized that I do belong to Him. I know He is with me. And when I'm scared, all I need is Him. It is then He sends His ministering servants in many different ways. It is then when He walks beside me or picks me up and carries me. There are times during this journey that I let fear come in and I feel panic, but peace slips in when I set my mind and heart on God and look to Him for who He is.

Yesterday was one of those peaceful days even though we had to say goodbye to Megan and her family and actually to Mindy and her family too. Megan and Mike are heading back to Michigan for a few weeks so that Michael can finish up the work he has to do to become a full-fledged

124

minister. They'll also finish packing up their Grand Rapids home and saying goodbye to friends. Mindy and her family are going to Eastern Iowa for a wedding reception for Sou's sister, one they all love much. So it is going to feel a little lonely this weekend. And yet I feel peaceful.

As I consider John 14:27, I know God is working in my heart. Jesus said, "Peace I leave with you; My peace I give to you" (NASB). Right now I am calm: I do belong to You. I know You are with me. Thank you for working Your peace in me. Thank you that I can rest assuredly in Your plan for me and there is nothing to fear in what comes from You. Thank you for those You send who speak in Your name. Thank you that I can have a peace that transcends all understanding.

I hope all of you, too, are feeling His peace even if you are going through trials in your life. If you are struggling to find peace, take time to read Psalm 29:11, Ephesians 2:17-18, and Philippians 4:7. I almost forgot to mention—I had a great treatment again yesterday. My blood pressure was down to normal! My counts were again excellent! Treatment went well. I once again zonked out during most of it, leaving my mom to fend for herself. I was extremely tired afterwards but that actually worked out quite well. I got home about 7:00, I fell asleep and was actually able to sleep the whole night, allowing me to get up very refreshed this morning. Thanks to all of you—for all you do for me.

In His Name.

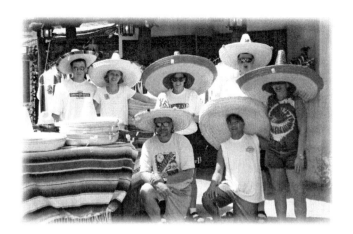

July/August 2007

Tuesday, July 3, 2007 9:08 a.m.

Good Morning,

Last evening I spent a good amount of time in my gardens. There were a few weeds to be pulled, some annuals to cut back, a little dead-heading to be done, and of course, the never-ending watering. Jerry usually does the watering—for a few different reasons. One, he thinks he does a better job than I; two, he thinks it tires me out too much (isn't he sweet?); and three, he likes it. He's been extra busy at work, so I've done the watering the past few days. We have a lot of plants around our yard so it takes a bit of time to fill their thirsty vessels. As I was nurturing my flowers, straightening some, adding some dirt here and there, pulling out dead leaves, adding a little weed killer or fertilizer where it was necessary, it reminded me much of our Christian life. Right now many of my flowers would have died without the tender, loving care we are giving them. They need constant attention, constant nurturing. So do we. As Christians we need constantly to take in the things that make us grow in our Christian life. We need to be nurtured. It doesn't work for us to live in isolation and grow. We need God's Word, a strong support system, good literature, inspirational speakers, and a time to reflect, to make our "garden" a beautiful place. We can only grow straight and tall and produce beauty if we take the time to feed and fertilize. My garden is beautiful right now. The lilies are vibrant, the meadow sage is ravishing in its second bloom, the balloon flowers are bursting forth color. That's the way we should be too—vibrant, ravishing, and colorful. I hope each of you enjoys the color in your life today, the color that comes from being nurtured in God's Word.

"May God himself, the God of peace, sanctify you through and through. May your whole spirit, soul and body be kept blameless at the coming of our Lord Jesus Christ" (I Thessalonians 5:23).

I've been extra busy the past few days. I am finishing up a summer course from USD and have almost completed one of the courses from last spring that I needed to finish. It feels good to be getting things completed. But along with a great sense of accomplishment comes extra fatigue. It's been difficult to deal with fatigue. When I study hard, I become completely exhausted. But besides that, I am feeling well. Each day I continue to have sore throats, but that is just another side effect of the medicine. So far I'm feeling good enough that I'm sure I'll be able to complete this series. Already on Thursday I will receive the last treatment of the first of the three. I'm thankful that I can continue on this drug.

Again I want to thank all for your prayers and other encouraging displays of kindness. Jerry finished up a casserole from a friend last night, and I've been enjoying two beautiful bouquets of flowers that I received. What a blessing to have support! Have a good day.

Wednesday, July 4, 2007 11:27 p.m.

Today we drove up to the lakes, unloaded our bikes, and rode around a good part of the west side of Okoboji. There are some nice rolling hills if you stay on Lakeshore Drive, hills that can make the novice biker's brow sweat and heart beat. It felt good to get some good exercise and we enjoyed being outdoors. Later we went for a drive around the lakes. Jerry loves to drive and "tour" the area. I don't. But since it was a holiday and I felt really generous today, I agreed to the ride. We looked at many houses and checked out some nice landscapes. We also rode by lots of fields, beautiful fields with crops that looked very healthy. Both of us remembered the old saying "knee high by the fourth" and had to laugh at that old saying. It surely didn't stand true today. The corn we saw today was over our heads and some was already tasseling. Even though I grew up as a farm girl, I don't know much about the farm, but I do know enough to understand that a lot has been invested into making corn mature faster and produce more.

That's what it takes in our lives too. Whatever we invest in, grows. It may be good things; it may be not so good things. It's important that we reflect on our lives and check our investments. Are we investing in other people or ourselves? Are we investing in material or spiritual things? Are we putting work into building God's kingdom or our own? I don't mean to judge people because I don't know where their investments lie, but as we rode around the lake tonight, I couldn't help but think of all the time and money spent on boats and houses and cars and entertainment. It's not that these things are bad in themselves, but if it's our only investment, we're laying up treasures "where moth and rust destroy and thieves break in to steal" (Matthew 6:19). God asks us to "store up for ourselves treasures in heaven" (vs. 20). Storing up treasures isn't limited to money; it includes all of our acts of obedience to God; even our intentions should seek the fulfillment of God's purposes in all we do. It's always good for us to check our investments.

Tomorrow I hope to get the last dose of chemo in this first of the next series. How does that sound for complicated? To put it simpler, I'll have my last of the infusions of this set of three. Next week I'll have a free week then I'll begin the second set of three. Dr. Krie hopes I can have three of these series and then we'll see what is next. I'm just praying that once again my counts will be good. I'm thankful that I've been able to have every treatment that has been planned so far and that I can still tolerate the side effects. I hope you had a wonderful holiday and enjoy a good day back at work. In Him.

Friday, July 6, 2007 12:42 a.m.

Hello dear friends,

I'm full of energy and I'm not quite sure what to do with it all. Jerry keeps telling me to sit down and rest, but I can't, so I'm glad he fell asleep. Today I had another great treatment. My counts were again very good and my blood pressure is staying down. I had a great nap during my treatment so time went fast. They woke me at 12:00 and told me I was finished, but I wasn't ready to wake up so I asked if they could wake me in a half hour. They tried thirty minutes later and I asked for one more half hour. It is amazing how much better I feel if I can sleep the Benadryl off rather than just leave when I'm finished. I think that is part of the reason I feel so energized tonight. I am thankful that I can continue with treatments on schedule.

A while back I mentioned to my friend Marlys Vander Pol that I was going to make sure I took time to read the book *Velvet Elvis* (by Rob Bell) this summer. She remarked that she was reading it right now and thought I would like it. Well, within a few days I received a copy of it from her in the mail. Thanks, Marlys; I love the book! While I was awake today, I re-read one of the most intriguing chapters titled "Tassels." The title is referring to the tassels (tzitzit) that many Jewish people tied to their garments. The book of Numbers gives specific directions of how to make the tassels, along with the command to look at them so the people would remember God's commands. Bell makes great connections between the Old and New Testament, ending with the story of the woman who touched Jesus' garment, believing she would be healed. He then tells her, "Go in peace." Go in shalom. When I was young we used to sing the song, "Shalom, My Friend." Peace my friend.

Over the last few years, especially after reading Syd Hielema's work, and now Rob Bell's book, I've come to see shalom as something that is much deeper than just peace, the absence of conflict. "Shalom is the presence of the goodness of God. It's the presence of wholeness, completeness." So when we are commanded to practice or "do" shalom, it involves living in complete harmony with God—in body, soul, spirit, mind and emotions—all of us. Wow! That means that everything I do, think, and say has to lead me to be more and more the kind of person God has made me to be. What a command! Bell says that Jesus' death on the cross is more than an act of forgiveness; it also includes "the on-going work of the cross in our hearts and minds and souls and lives. There is the on-going need to return to the cross to be reminded of our brokenness and dependence on God." I know I for one often take God's gift of forgiveness for granted. I have to see it in a much bigger picture than just me; it is about God. It is about a God who made me and wants me to be a healthy, whole, life-giving person who lives my life in shalom.

"Shalom, my friend, shalom, my friend, shalom, shalom . . . ." May you too live in the shalom that God intended. Peace.

Monday, July 9, 2007 2:37 p.m.

On Friday evening we went with Mindy, Sou, the boys and my parents to Lake Pahoja. It was a beautiful evening. We had fun grilling hot dogs, making smores, playing ball, and swinging on the swings. Miles, the one-year-old, had me gasping over and over as he finagled himself up the steps of the slide. I couldn't believe how he could hang and twist and pull to get where he wanted to go. Kobi and Bailey had a great time playing ball with grandpa. On the way home Bailey and I were sitting in the back seat of the Suburban when he began to sing a song. He said to me, "That's a song that Kobi sang at the Christmas program." He sang it again and this time I listened closer to the words he was singing. "Don't tell it on the mountains, over the hills and everywhere . . . ." Mindy was listening and she said, "No, Bailey. It isn't don't, it's go." There was no convincing Bailey. As we all sang the song (over and over), Bailey continued to sing "Don't." That's how, in his mind, the song was supposed to go.

I find that happening in my life too. I don't always get things right, not because I don't want to but because of immaturity or a poor understanding. I think back over the years at my spiritual development, and even though I still have much to learn, I can see where I have grown from misunderstandings or inaccurate beliefs that I had when I was young. I'm thankful for the truth of God's Word, truth that doesn't change. But that doesn't mean that my understanding of God's Word isn't dynamic, constantly changing. A guest minister we had years ago reminded us that if our spiritual development was the same as it was five years before, or three years, or even one year, then we weren't growing. He said we weren't looking deep enough into the scriptures and challenging ourselves to understand God better. I've thought about that a lot over the years. It's something that continually challenges me to read and study God's Word and find what God wants me to understand about Him. The Jewish rabbis would sometimes put honey on the fingers of their students and have them taste it, reminding them that God's Word is like the taste of honey on the tongue—delicious, sweet!

It is often hard for me to get going in the morning so it is sometimes tempting to sleep in or at least just laze around until I have more energy. Yesterday morning was like that. I felt like staying home. Church is sometimes an emotional place for me. Talking to people, singing songs, hearing scripture, any of those things can bring me to tears quite easily. But I went and as usual was tremendously blessed. We had a great challenge through the message, friends from out of town were in church and it was good to talk to them, and I was again reminded by so many people that they were praying for me. Thank you to all of you who pray for me. Every day I feel your prayers. Every day I'm touched by your willingness to pray for me. It is humbling. Have a good week.

Tuesday, July 10, 2007 10:29 a.m.

Good Morning,

I'm a little late this morning. I finally found sleep and just couldn't wake up this morning.

A few years ago when I was still teaching in the elementary classroom, my beautician decided to give me a new hairdo. I went to school the next day, eager to see if the students noticed. I didn't have to wait long. As I was walking down the hall to supervise first recess duty, little Jordan joined me and said, "Mrs. Bosma, are you having a bad hair day?" Ooooh-stab #1. Only a few minutes later another student looked down the hallway and said to the teacher he was walking with, "What happened to Mrs. Bosma; did she get up on the wrong side of bed?" Ooooh-stab #2. Before anyone else could comment, I pulled my hair back into a ponytail for the rest of the day.

What does it mean to get up on the wrong side of bed? To this student, it must have meant I didn't have enough time to do my hair, at least not properly. But usually it means that we start our day "out-of-sorts." It means that we're grumpy. Our guest minister on Sunday told us of research that says most children don't get up "on the wrong side of bed."

They awake worry free and happy. It's adults who begin their day with burdens and worries and discontent. Yes, many of us have many things that concern us. It might be finances; it might be health; it might be family worries. Proverbs 15:15b says, " . . . but the cheerful heart has a continual feast." Things may not always go as we planned or hoped; we can't change that, but we can choose how we respond. If we fill our thoughts with things that are true, pure, right, admirable (Philippians 4:8), we can have a right attitude even when we are in tough situations. God loves a cheerful heart. Live your life with a continual feast of happiness.

And speaking of happiness, yesterday was one of those days that was filled with happiness. To begin with, the day started too early. I had a difficult time sleeping because of all the different pains in my feet. That may sound strange but this is how it was—I have an infected sore from scratching open a rash that developed on my right foot; I have a new rash on the other side of that foot, and the tingling on the bottom of my feet was about the worst it has ever been. As I was about to fall asleep, a new pain would hit. I tried more lotions and creams. So when 7:00 a.m. rolled around, I wasn't ready to get up. That doesn't sound like happiness does it. Jerry had a meeting in Omaha so I decided to ride along and take a jog over to USD in Vermillion to check on the status of my program. While I was there I found out that a test I took to enter the Ed.D. program was high enough for me to be accepted. What a huge relief!

In Omaha, I was able to visit with one of our good friends, Jeff Osler. When I got home there was another card of encouragement from Aunt Lucy, a journal entry from Jaiden, and then I talked to Megan and she told me that today she was in leadership training with two students I had had in class and had traveled with to Nicaragua. It is exciting to think of the impact these young lives will have in God's kingdom. Happiness comes in many different ways and from many different things. I guess that's what makes a feast! I hope you experience a feast today. In Him.

Wednesday, July 11, 2007 9:21 a.m.
Hello,

It's another one of those days when I woke up fatigued—just a continuation from yesterday, I guess. I have much work I want to get finished today but we'll see how that goes. I did get through a few lessons on my on-line course yesterday and I hope to get some more done today. I also want to take time to see Kobi and Bailey's last t-ball game. So I'm not writing much this morning—I'll try to get back later. Thanks for keeping me in your prayers.

Thursday, July 12, 2007 12:52 a.m.

Psalm 150 is one of my favorite Psalms. It's a closing hymn of praise, like a doxology. Over the past few years this Psalm has become our praise to God when we arrive in Cary with the serve team. Just after arrival, we read this Psalm and then paraphrase it to praise God for our specific joys. Today I feel this Psalm welling up in me: "Praise God in his sanctuary; praise him in his mighty heavens. Praise him for his acts of power; praise him for his surpassing greatness. Praise him with the sounding of the trumpet, praise him with the harp and lyre, praise him with tambourine and dancing, praise him with strings and flute, praise him with the clash of cymbals, praise him with resounding cymbals. Let everything that has breath praise the Lord. Praise the Lord."

Can you imagine the beautiful and joyous sound put out by all these instruments? That's what our lives should be like. Some of us may have more natural musical ability than others, but that doesn't make a difference. Jerry has a difficult time carrying a tune and even more difficulty singing and clapping to the beat. (Just ask the kids who have gone with us to Cary.) The kids sometimes give him a hard time about his musical talents, but that never deters him from singing from his heart and often leading "the pack" during our praise time.

If we think about it, all of us have much to praise God for. When I consider His surpassing greatness and power, I can say "Praise God!"

I praise God for my family. I praise Him for great friends.
I praise Him for my colleagues who always encourage me.
I praise God for a great department secretary and work study, for the help they've given me.
I praise God for conversations with friends who were back at Dordt for the grad ed. program.
I praise Him for giving me more energy and for less pain in my feet and nose.
I praise Him for great medical care.
I praise Him for giving me life and the opportunity to live!
I praise Him for all the prayers that have been offered on my behalf. Praise the Lord!

Friday, July 13, 2007 2:24 a.m.

My dear friends,

I've been trying to sleep for a few hours, and it's not working so I decided I could just as well get up and write. Today was a reminder to me that I must have many prayer warriors out there. I felt the best I have felt in a long time. I had "coffee" with my friend Doris this morning, something I looked forward to doing. After I got home, I went to work on my on-line course and I worked until early this evening, finishing up all the chapter questions and quizzes. What a great feeling! I had so much ambition that I made a pretty good dinner for Jerry. My cousin Bryan stopped over so we invited him to stay too. It felt good to be able to work the whole day without feeling too fatigued. Unfortunately, as you can see by this post, my ambition has lasted into the wee hours. All of this is what got me to think about prayer. I don't know how many people pray for me, but it is probably more than I realize, and I want to thank you very much. Some of you have reminded me that you pray for me when I can't. Thank you! Some of you have told me that you pray for me every day. Thank you! God has worked in many of your hearts to do this and once again, all I can say is that I am very humbled and thankful.

These verses have come to me often: "Be joyful in hope, patient in affliction, faithful in prayer"(Romans 12:12). "Do not be anxious about anything, but in everything, by prayer and petition, with thanksgiving, present your requests to God" (Philippians 4:6). "And the prayer offered in faith will make the sick person well" (James 5:15). The NIV commentary says that the prayer offered in faith refers to the faith of the people who are praying. Our prayers are subject to God's will. But our prayers are part of the healing process. That may be why God often waits for our prayers before intervening to heal a person.

"For the eyes of the Lord are on the righteous and his ears are attentive to their prayer" (I Peter 3:12). "If you believe, you will receive whatever you ask for in prayer"(Matthew 21:22). The commentary says this isn't a guarantee we will get what we ask for. To be answered, our requests must be in line with God's will, but God does move our hearts to pray.

There is no substitute for prayer. I thank God for putting it in your heart to pray! In Him.

Monday, July 16, 2007 9:13 a.m.

Good Morning dear friends,

Sundays are a blessing and yesterday was no different. Our grandsons had stayed overnight, so we woke up to a busy and happy house. I had to go to church early to go over some music for the morning service, so Jerry was in charge of the boys. We never know what to expect when he's in charge! He did a great job. He enjoyed breakfast with them on the deck, dressed the boys for church and then braved sitting alone with them in church. That didn't last too long. He caught the eye of Jaleesa, one of our young friends, and gave her a look of desperation. She caught on and came and sat by him. We celebrated communion and that, along with a powerful sermon, was very moving. Catherine and I played which enriches the service for me. As we contemplate the texts and the parts of worship, we look for songs that will complement and enhance the service, and that in turn makes the service richer for me. I'm very thankful for corporate worship where God's people come together to praise and glorify Him.

But even with all the joy of the weekend, there still exists nagging thoughts, those what ifs. What if I don't see the boys? What if I can't help Jerry with . . . ? What if I can't handle the schedule of classes this fall?

In reality the cancer is gone now, but it is also very real that it could return. That is obvious to me when I hear of people who seem to "beat" their cancer only to have it return a short time later. Here comes another what if—what if that happens to me? I know the right answer in my head; God is in control and He will walk beside me and carry me, whatever the path. But convincing my heart isn't always easy. In Isaiah 49:16 we read: "See, I have engraved you on the palms of my hands." What a comfort to know that even when I worry, even when I fear, God has my name written on the palm of His hand and He will not let me go. He has your name there too. I'll continue to pray that He will help me see and believe His powerful ways. In Him.

Wednesday, July 18, 2007 3:20 a.m.

Dear friends,

Yesterday I met with Dr. Krie and had the first of the second series of treatments. I thought my appointment was on Thursday, but a call from Dr. Krie's office alerted me to my appointment. If I don't take care with my appointment cards, I completely forget when my next appointment is. For a short time after treatments, I find I can't depend on my memory. The nurses call it "chemo brain" or the effects of a strong dose of Benadryl. I'm not sure. After my treatment, my sister Marcia met me at the mall to do a little shopping. I loved shopping with her, but even more, I love how she helped me find my car in the parking lot. It took us 15 minutes riding around in her car. Can you imagine how long it would have taken me if I would have had to walk? I can attribute this "car loss" to my recent chemo treatment or to my being a Cleveringa. I think my Cleveringa cousins know which it is.

My counts were excellent again today. I had a complete range of tests done, visited with Dr. Krie and had a full infusion treatment. I again had a good nap that continued for about an hour after my treatment. The nurses are kind to let me sleep until I'm ready to wake up.

After a little shopping, Marcia and I had dinner together and talked about life, its trials and joys. (I don't know if I've ever mentioned that she is finished with chemo and radiation and is now taking a pill for the next five years. She appears to be cancer free and hopes the pill will keep her free.) We talked about my visit with Dr. Krie, about the statistics, about the future, and about our trip this weekend to Grand Rapids (more about that later). We talked about the half empty/half full paradigm, how in life you can look at what happens as a glass half empty or half full. How you see the glass depends on your point of view. If you see the glass as half full, you are probably an optimist. If you see it as half empty, you are probably a pessimist. I have to admit, I do occasionally fall into the half empty category. Not that I want to, but, especially when I'm fatigued, it happens. I know I have to be realistic, but I also know that God wants me to use every day to honor and glorify Him and I can't do that when my glass is half empty.

When you look at scripture, you can easily see how God wants us to view life.

Look at these verses: Psalm 42:5: "Why are you so downcast, O my soul? Why so disturbed within me? Put your hope in God, for I will yet praise him, my Savior and my God." And at Psalm 62:5: "Find rest, O my soul, in God alone; my hope comes from him. He alone is my fortress, I will not be shaken. My salvation and my honor depend on God, he is my mighty rock, my refuge." Psalm 147:11 adds this: "The Lord delights in those who fear him, who put their hope in his unfailing love."

When we trust in God, put our hope in Him as our rock and fortress, our attitude on life changes. No longer are we held hostage by the trials in our life. When we look, we see God's goodness, faithfulness, and love. When we look to God, we focus on His ability rather than our own. That's when we praise Him for all of life's journeys! I hope you see your life as a half full glass. In Him.

Thursday, July 19, 2007 12:04 a.m.

Hello friends,

Fireflies. Those little bugs that have us curious about their glow. Jerry and I often sit on our deck late in the evening and watch the little bugs as they flitter here and there around our house. We watch them glow as they fly in the grass. Our grandchildren love the fireflies too. They squeal with delight as they chase them and try to capture them so they can put them in their bug houses. When our own children were young, we used to play a game. It went like this—when the fireflies hit the windshield, we would make guesses as to how long the firefly would glow. We discovered that fireflies could glow from between a few seconds to several minutes. This little game may not sound too exciting to you, but it helped pass time as we traveled.

It's the glow that intrigues me. What makes them glow? Why do they glow? A quick search on the Internet will give you all the information you need to know about fireflies. A quick search of the Bible tells us that we are to glow too. Our reason for glowing is different than the fireflies but just as important. The fireflies glow so that they can find a mate and reproduce. We glow so that we can demonstrate our love for Christ and in turn show others who Christ is. In a way we want to reproduce who Christ was as he walked on earth. Our hearts, dead to sin, need a heart change to do this. When that happens we can begin to look like Christ. How often do we glow in our life? How often do we give a good representation of Christ?

As I rode home from my chemo treatment this week, I caught a piece of David Jeremiah's message. He told of a conversation he had with a non-Christian. This person said he didn't want to become a Christian because of the behavior he observed in Christians. He didn't give examples, but I could think of quite a few: language that isn't wholesome or uplifting, butting in lines or line hopping so we can be first, slander or gossip, cheating, little "white" lies, conceit, gambling, a diet of raunchy movies, raw or degrading jokes, and the list goes on.

Isaiah 60:1 reads: "Arise, shine for your light has come, and the glory of the LORD rises upon you." And Matthew 5:14-16: "You are the light of the world. A city on a hill cannot be hidden. Neither do people light a lamp and put it under a bowl. Instead they put it on its stand, and it gives light to everyone in the house. In the same way, let your light shine before men, that they may see your good deeds and praise your Father in heaven."

If we live for Christ, we will glow. Just as we are intrigued with the fireflies' glow, others will notice our glow and we hope grow in Christ.

My day went as I expected it would. After a sleepless night, I didn't have much energy today. I had hoped to get a big paper finished, but I couldn't concentrate. I did get a bedroom cleaned so I felt that I accomplished something. I'm having more nausea after this treatment. Dr. Krie said that symptoms will probably worsen as treatments continue. I have some medication that I hope will help.

Thanks much for all your prayers and ways that you continue to encourage me. Each day I am amazed by your thoughtfulness and care. I wish I could thank every one of you in person but since I can't, I hope you read this and feel appreciated. Have a good day!

Wednesday, July 25, 2007 10:23 a.m.
Dear friends,

Wow! It's been a long time since I posted on my site. We left on Friday for Michigan and returned home on Monday night. I left for Sioux Falls early Tuesday morning for a treatment so it's been busy. We had a wonderful time in Michigan. True to fashion, Megan had plans for some Western Michigan fun on Saturday. We first went blueberry picking (h-m-m-m delicious) and then we traveled on to Lake Michigan. It wasn't swimming weather but the sights were great. On Sunday we celebrated Michael's installation into the ministry. Along with a very meaningful service (planned by Michael), the installation was especially touching for us. The laying on of hands was powerful and very moving. This was Michael's last step so he is now a full-fledged minister. It was also the last thing that kept them in Michigan, so before we left, we packed most of their things into a trailer to take to Iowa. Most of the Nigerian boxes are marked and ready to go so they will be ready to go to the airport on August 15 and the rest will be put into storage until they return in what they predict right now to be in five years. They've been sorting and packing for months so now that is off their mind too.

Thinking of their packing reminded me of life. Each of us packs many things into our life—stuff, activities, thoughts, actions. It seems we acquire quite a bunch of "stuff" that is unnecessary and sometimes even unhealthy. It would be good for each of us to take time out and sort through that "stuff" and see what needs to stay and what has to go. I'm afraid we would all find plenty of "stuff" that we should get rid of. That takes time, time to "Be still," time to reflect, time to glorify. We heard a great sermon on Sunday on the meaning of glorify—in a nutshell, it constitutes all the things we do in our life. I need to take more time each day to contemplate what I'm storing up. II Corinthians 4:7-12 says, "But we have this treasure in jars of clay to show that this all-surpassing power is from God and not from us. We are hard pressed on every side, but not crushed; perplexed, but not in despair; persecuted, but not abandoned,; struck down but not destroyed. We always carry around in our body the death of Jesus, so that the life of Jesus may also be revealed in our body. For we who are alive are always being given over to death for Jesus' sake, so that his life may be at work in you." Our "jars of clay" are fragile and can be easily damaged or destroyed, but what's inside those jars are contents that can never be destroyed and can be used for powerful work for the kingdom. Michael and Megan's work of sorting through their personal things was a good reminder for me to sort.

My treatment went well again yesterday. One thing I am finding is that nothing is consistent in this business of treatments. Just when I think I have a pattern figured out, things change. I again felt quite good after my treatment, but fatigue and nausea quickly set in. The last few times I've been wide awake until early the next morning, but this time I went into a tight sleep until early morning and that's when I became wide awake. So I guess I have to be ready for anything. I'm very thankful for very little pain in my fingers and toes, at least for today. I'm feeling energized and ready to work, so I'd better get at it while I'm feeling like it.

Thank you once again for all your prayers and kind deeds. Michael, Megan and the kids will be traveling to Iowa today so if you find a minute, please pray for safe travel. They've made many Iowa trips and each one has been blessed with safety.

Enjoy the warmth while you pray for rain.

Thursday, July 26, 2007 10:38 a.m.

Good Morning,

Just a quick note—Michael and Megan arrived late yesterday afternoon—safe once again. We are thankful for safety as they travel. We are leaving in a few minutes for a little vacation with the kids. A wonderful friend has lent us their home on West Okoboji for the weekend. We are grateful for this opportunity and are looking forward to spending some quiet, relaxing time with our whole family. Of course, the grandkids may have different ideas. God surely does provide through friends and family.

I'm thankful that my hands and feet are feeling fine. Last week I wasn't sure I would be able to keep up this treatment for another month and a half, but for now it looks like it's possible. Please keep praying that this can happen. Thanks again for your prayers and all the other many things you do to encourage not only me, but our whole family. In Him.

Wednesday, August 1, 2007 9:00 p.m.

Hello dear friends,

Time has flown. It has been almost a week since I've written on my site. Adding four more people to a house (Michael, Megan, Amira, and Nico arrived on Wednesday), going on vacation, and getting a treatment have all added to this. We are thoroughly enjoying our full house; vacation was absolutely fantastic, and treatment went well.

About our vacation—we spent five wonderful days on West Okoboji enjoying our grandkids and their parents, the lake, and the facilities. We swam, boated, played, watched a couple of plays, and enjoyed good home-cooked meals and dining out. We loved listening to the squeals of the grandkids as they sat in the front of the boat and felt the water as it sprayed on them. It was fun to watch their expressions as they observed the characters act in Peter Pan. We enjoyed all the activity, but we also enjoyed being surrounded by a beautiful environment. It was amazing to wake up each morning, rise up on one elbow, look out the west windows and then see the sun reflecting on the smooth water. If I looked out the windows on the right side of the bedroom, I could see the trees reflected in the clear blue water. What a gorgeous sight 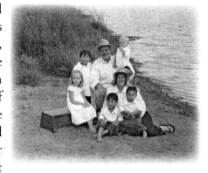 to set the tone for the day! Soon the tranquility of the lake was destroyed by the boaters, but the memory of the early morning beauty lingered on. With this memory tucked in my heart and mind, it was difficult to let anything ruin my day.

God created a beautiful world and even though we continue to ruin it and wear down that beauty, there is still much to enjoy. Sometimes it is difficult to slow down and see it. Each day we rush around trying to accomplish all the work before us, and we fail to be revived and inspired by all that surrounds us, things that remind us of who God is and how He cares for us. God created a functional world that helps sustain life. We were reminded of that as we drove past the bean, corn, wheat, and sorghum fields. But He also created a great, big, beautiful world for us to enjoy, which is exactly what we did this weekend. We took time to enjoy the rising and setting of the sun, the distinct and different characteristics of our grandchildren, the talents of the actors, the delicious taste of a variety of foods, funny stories, the smooth, quiet night water, the beautiful house in which we stayed, finding fish as they swam under the dock, getting caught in seaweed, reading, and much more. We also enjoyed the people God has put in our lives—our family and also the friends with whom we were able to visit. We truly were blessed by this time away and we thank our dear friends from Dordt for their gracious offer of letting us use their house which made all of this possible. What a gift. These memories will stay with us forever. We will forever treasure our opportunity to strengthen family ties and enjoy God's creation. It was a poignant reminder for all of us to continue to look for God's blessings throughout each and every day. (I'm going to try sending this post in two postings.)

Wednesday, August 1, 2007 9:02 p.m.

(Continued . . .)Yesterday was my last treatment in the second set of the second series. I have one more set to go to finish out the second series. My counts were again very good although my white count keeps slipping. It is now in the low category. My infusion nurse told me I should not eat raw fruits and vegetables because of the bugs that remain on them, even after washing. Usually your white cells are able to fight off these bugs, but right now my body might not be able to. She also warned me about touching my flowers and digging in the dirt where I can pick up bugs. I guess I'll finally get some use out of the garden gloves that Jerry insists I use. Dr. Krie stopped in to visit today while I was getting treatment and we talked over the plan for the next few months. She thinks I should plan on going for one more series in August and then take a month off. At first I was skeptical of taking that much time off treatment, but with much assurance from her, she convinced me. It will be wonderful to have the whole month of September off so that I can teach without having to worry about chemo treatments. Of course, I'll have to have a CT scan before this all happens to make sure no cancer is growing now. I asked her about the possibility of the cancer returning during the month off and she said it's possible but we'll start treatment again and they should be able to take care of it again. Of course, there is always the possibility that it won't come back that quickly, which is what we will be praying for. Another reason to rely on God and trust Him to lead us on this journey.

I have a few tee-shirts that say, "Life is good" and I wear them because I believe it is good. It is good because God runs it, not from afar, but right down here among His people. Life is good, as these texts remind us: Psalm 100:5: "For the LORD is good and his love endures forever; his faithfulness continues through all generations." Psalm 34:8: "Taste and see that the Lord is good; blessed is the man who takes refuge in him."

Look for God in the usual and in the unusual. Enjoy what He has given you.

Sunday, August 19, 2007 10:19 p.m.

Dear friends,

Wow! What a sabbatical—it wasn't seven years, but I have been away from this site for a long time. Even though it was a great three weeks, it was also exhausting. It was wonderful to be able to spend time with Michael, Megan, Nico and Amira along with Mindy and Sou and their boys, but it did keep me busy and pretty exhausted. Michael and Megan left Wednesday and I think I slept every spare minute for the next three days.

I hardly know where to begin so I think I'll take time in this journal to tell you about what's going on with my health. I had a doctor's appointment on Thursday, the day after Mike and Megan left. Mindy went with me—I don't like to go to a doctor's appointment by myself. I did the normal, routine things—had blood drawn, temperature taken, blood pressure checked. All the time I'm thinking—I sure hope my counts are all okay so I can have a treatment. Well, all my counts were okay but after lots of questions from Dr. Krie, she decided that she should hold off on more treatments for a month. I've developed neuropathy which is a numbing and tingling in my fingers and toes. I've had this pain for the last few months, but it has really increased the past month. Jerry has been a dear through all of this. Each night he diligently rubs a special lotion on my feet. The lotion helps lessen the pain but so far we haven't found anything that takes the pain away. Permanent damage can result if the nerves become too damaged, plus (a long story made short) it can limit our chemo options later. So I have a month off which I am very ready for—no treatment, no traveling, no time spent sitting in the infusion room (although I will miss all my friends and nurses at the infusion center).

On September 20 I will have another PET scan which will help Dr. Krie decide what will happen next. At my last appointment she reminded me that there is no cookie-cutter answer or a single recipe for cancer. Each case is very individual and is treated as such, but we do have some ideas about what the future could look like. If the scan shows no cancer growth, I could go on a low dose of chemo and I would have periodic scans to watch for new growth; or if cancer does show up after the month off from treatment, I could possibly go back on the treatment I was on, or maybe Dr. Krie will suggest another chemo, depending on the advancement or decrease of the neuropathy. I've been told that chemo stays in your body for awhile so I know that one month off isn't going to give me all of my energy back, but I'm hoping some of the fatigue will decrease.

Thanks for all the continued prayers and expressions of encouragement. I very much appreciate the suggestions that some of you send my way. Please join us in prayer this month as we pray for my lungs to stay clear and for renewed energy. God has blessed us the past month by letting us spend much time with family and friends, and we are grateful. I have much more to write but I'll save it for a later day. I promise I won't stay away so long again. In Him.

Tuesday, August 21, 2007 11:48 p.m.

Dear friends,

As many of you know, Michael, Megan, Amira and Nico left last week for Abuja, Nigeria. We had much to do before they left and enjoyed them so much that we didn't really concentrate on their leaving until the very end. But eventually we had to face the fact that they were going to travel half-way around the world and be gone from the U.S. for at least two years. The goodbye at the airport was really difficult. I can still see Amira's sad little face with tears streaming down her cheeks. Saying goodbye to one's grandchildren is very difficult. Thankfully, within a little over 24 hours we heard from them—they were already settled into their new home. On their way to the Daniel Center where they will be living, Amira, who had been scanning the countryside as they rode, announced, "I think I'm going to like this place!" Those were great words to hear. Granted it is early and I'm sure she'll have some hard days ahead of her, but attitude is everything and hearing her voice her approval of her new country was encouraging.

Attitude is a big part of life. Research done with cancer patients reveals that those who have a positive attitude live longer. That's amazing to me. We do have a choice of how we can look at things, negatively or positively. How do we get that positive attitude? Not by our own power, but by the grace of God. What a gift! James 1:17 says, "Every good and perfect gift is from above, coming down from the Father of the heavenly lights, who does not change like the shifting shadows." God's grace helps us to embrace our circumstances with peace and confidence. I thank God for giving me what I need when I need it, and I'm thankful that He gave Amira a feeling of belonging as she rode down the new streets in her new city.

I continue to be amazed by those of you who remember me, and I know that I don't have a clue of how many are praying for me. Thank you very much. Prayer is powerful. I'm feeling relief in my feet and some in my fingers. Sometimes I deduce things without medical proof, but it seems my body aches more the past week, and I believe it is due to not having the premeds that I got before earlier treatments. I've found that there are other drugs to help that too. Soon I'll be a pro on medications. Some of you are beginning school tomorrow; I'm praying (whether you are a student or a teacher) that you have a wonderful beginning to an exciting year of discovering talents and exploring God's wonderful world. School, what a great place to be! I have one more week to get my act together and be prepared for classes. In Him.

Thursday, August 23, 2007 9:38 p.m.

Hello friends,

Rainy days are always good days for nostalgia. Listening to the pitter-patter of the rain on our skylight brought me back to rainy days when I was a kid. My twin sister and I never liked those days. We used to chant a few sayings when we were cooped up in the house. One went like this, "Rain, rain go away, come again another day." We, of course, at that young age, didn't think of the benefit of rain but rather we were concerned about not being able to ride horse or play in the sandbox. There was another little ditty that went something like this: "It's raining; it's pouring; the old man is snoring. He bumped his head on a baby bed and couldn't get up the next morning." I'm not sure but I think it meant that someone upstairs was out of commission and couldn't stop the rain. We only said the second ditty a few times, because as soon as my mom heard it, she gave us a stern warning and called it *spotten*. (For those of you who aren't Dutch, the word means poking fun of God.) As I said, my mom put a quick stop to us saying this little phrase, but it has stuck with me all these years. Isn't that true of negative words, phrases or thoughts that we have heard over the years? Even though we would like to get rid of them, those things often lurk in the back of our minds, coming to the forefront when we are angry, upset, anxious or troubled. That is why Philippians 4:8 is important to remember: "Finally, brothers, whatever is true, whatever is noble, whatever is right, whatever is pure, whatever is lovely, whatever is admirable—if anything is excellent or praiseworthy— think about such things." What we put in our minds comes out in our words and actions. But we find comfort in verse 7 which says, "And the peace of God, which transcends all understanding, will guard your hearts and minds in Christ Jesus."

In elementary school we used to sing the song "Input, Output, What Goes In, Must Come Out." After we sang the song we would talk about the kinds of things that were good to put in our minds and the kinds of things that were dangerous. Students often mentioned the importance of being discerning with television, books, conversations, choice of language, movies, and magazines. It remains important for us as adults to continue to discern and choose things that fill our minds with wholesome things. It takes practice, encouragement from others, staying in God's Word, and prayer. When what "comes out" is wholesome, we are standing stones that reflect Christ.

As far as my health goes, I'm still struggling with fatigue. It seems I can have good energy one day and then the next day I'm zapped. Sometimes on those days I'm very sleepy, but sometimes it results in no ambition. My head feels groggy and it is really hard to get motivated to do anything. I cherish your prayers for renewed energy. I have less than one week before classes begin, and I do want to be prepared and ready for my students. Thanks and love to you all.

Sunday, August 26, 2007 10:29 p.m.

Dear friends,

Today we helped the Schreur family celebrate the adoption of their new daughter. It was a celebration filled with joy as we celebrated Chyann joining their family. It was also a reminder of God's faithfulness that has been shown to Nate and Cath over the past seven years. Chyann is a lovely five-year-old who is very happy to be a part of her new family. We love her already and are thrilled for Nate and Catherine.

Before we ate lunch today at noon, Cath read a passage that has come to mean a lot to them over the past few years as they have waited patiently for a child. It's odd how one passage can mean different things to different people who are dealing with different situations. Lamentations 3:22-24 is one text I have often looked at over the past few months. It has helped me cling to the promises of God's love and mercy. The passage reads: "Because of the LORD's great love we are not consumed, for his compassions never fail. They are new every morning; great is your faithfulness. I say to myself, 'The Lord is my portion; therefore I will wait on him.'" Nate and Cath prayed this prayer almost daily as they waited to see what God had in store for them.

As Cath read the passage, it reminded me how universal the Bible is. It was written years ago for a special group of people, and yet it has much meaning for all kinds of people in different situations today. What a fantastic book! I'm very thankful that we have the opportunity and privilege of reading it whenever we want to. I wonder how often we take this for granted.

I've again been reminded of my limitations. Yesterday was a busy day at Dordt. As faculty, we had a part in welcoming the new freshmen to the campus. It meant standing and talking a lot. After that we helped Kobi celebrate his sixth birthday at the Hull park. I came home extremely tired with every part of my body aching. After taking some medication and rolling restlessly in bed, I finally fell asleep. Days like that make me nervous about going back to a rigorous schedule at school this week. I guess I need to look to Lamentations 3 and believe that God in His faithfulness will see me through. Many people have assured me of their prayers. Thanks so much! Often I don't feel worthy of all the time people spend praying for me, but I guess it's not my worthiness but God's love that makes this all possible.

Have a wonderful week, filled with the assurance that our great, big, wonderful God is watching over all of us.

Tuesday, August 28, 2007 10:00 p.m.

Hello dear friends,

Remember the other day I when I talked about attitudes? Well today I heard a good story that connected to attitudes and I thought you might enjoy it too. This morning at breakfast Amira was dawdling at eating her cereal while she continued to tell Megan, "I don't want to go to school! I don't want to go to school!" Megan told her that sometimes we have to do things even when we don't want to. Elisha, their house help, was working in the kitchen so Megan thought she would elicit his help in changing Amira's attitude so she said, "Elisha, sometimes you do things, don't you, when you don't feel like it?" She was hoping he would buy into the conversation and convince Amira. He replied appropriately that, yes, he was expecting a very busy day and he was going to have to do things that he didn't feel like doing. Amira, our ever-thinking six-year-old responded, "Well then mom, why don't you give him the day off." I guess she thought that might give her the day off too. It didn't work! She had to go to school and she came home with a great big smile. Isn't it true; often when we have to do some things, it turns out that we enjoy them. Sometimes we have to put our mind to it. A good verse to keep in mind is Proverbs 15:15: "All the days of the oppressed are wretched, but the cheerful heart has a continual feast." Our attitudes show who we are. A famous saying says, "You can't always choose what happens to you, but you can choose your attitude toward each situation."

Today I've been struggling with my syllabi, something I've been working on for a long time. I couldn't put the finishing touches on them.

Then my friend Pat called, gave me some good advice and voila, I finished up two of them. It's a good thing too because tomorrow we begin classes. I'm very much looking forward to teaching and working with the students, but as I've said before, I'm very nervous about having the energy to do a good job. I love teaching and I have found that just being in my office, dealing with school things, has given me energy. I hope you will pray with me that I can accomplish all that is before me.

My health—the numbness in my feet has improved over the past week. As long as I don't stand on my feet for long periods of time, they feel almost normal. My finger tips are still quite numb, but I hope that will improve too. I'm enjoying the time off chemo. By the way, Dr. Krie told me that the Sioux Center hospital can now give me my treatments if I have to go back on Paxel and Avastin. Of course, I'm hoping and praying that my lungs stay clear so I don't need the "hard" chemo.

Once more, thanks for all your prayers. I am thankful for the assurance that He hears and responds. In Him.

Friday, August 31, 2007 12:06 a.m.

Dear friends,

I've just finished two days of teaching. I've met all my students and taught all my classes once. It was great to be in the classroom again. It's exciting and energizing to be around eager students as they look forward to the year. But I must say, some students looked more anxious than eager today. By the last class I taught today, most of them had received five syllabi (schedules) with all their assignments for the year. It's quite possible they've experienced information overload. Soon they'll settle in and learn to take one day at a time and the load won't look so overwhelming. As I dismissed my last class today, I thought of the day I received the news that I had cancer. I felt overwhelmed and scared. I was afraid of the future. Now here it is, more than six months later, and I'm back to teaching and, except for the fatigue, life is pretty normal. I'm thankful that I'm able to teach, enjoy my family and friends, love each day, and look forward to the future. Today was a good reminder of Isaiah 41:13: "For I am the LORD, your God, who takes hold of your right hand and says to you, Do not fear; I will help you." Through everything God's grip has held me fast. I hope you have felt His loving hands holding yours too.

Have a wonderful day, enjoying the beautiful fall weather.

SEPTEMBER-DECEMBER 2007

Sunday, September 2, 2007 11:11 p.m.

After spending almost every late afternoon and evening resting or sleeping, I decided it was time to break the habit and step out and do something different. I figured I could sleep on Saturday morning if I was tired. So our whole family (all who live here) went to the Western/Unity football game. We enjoyed brats and hot dogs at the tailgate party provided by Iowa State Bank, visiting with friends, watching our grandkids play on the sidelines, watching our friends Jaleesa and Erin cheer, and a little football. The weather was beautiful which made the whole evening even grander. I'd never gone to a high school football game so this was a new experience for me. One of the reasons I wanted to go was that I had six former fifth grade students playing on the team. It amazed me to see how much they had grown up and what good football players they were. Brennen was the QB, Kyle was named the most valuable player of the game by a radio station, and Nate, Adam, and Justin looked hot and sweaty when they came off the field so I assume they played hard which is what you need to do in any game. Jason must have been injured because he wasn't dressed for the game. I think back to the year I had those guys in class. They were wonderful kids and great students. These same athletes put on a musical and staged a pretty awesome wax museum.

But I remember in particular one thing they taught me. I was sitting by my desk looking over some last-minute lesson details and happened to catch a little of their conversation as they were hanging up their backpacks. I caught phrases like, "When I grow up, I'm going to play for the NFL" and "Not me, I want to play for the NBA. I'm going to . . . ." Lofty dreams. But more than that, it struck me, from what I was hearing, that none of them were imagining themselves working in God's kingdom right now. They were looking to the future—looking to the time when they were grown up and "punching a clock." I still remember the long talk we had that day (I wonder if any of them remember it) about how they were a part of God's kingdom now. They didn't have to wait until they were older—God's promises and the responsibilities of being a Christian belonged to them right now. Their responsibilities may look different than those of their parents, but they were just as important. I'll never forget the end of that year. The students' attitudes improved, as did their work. It was exciting to see. God expects all of us, whether young or old, to honor and praise Him in our work, and yes, in our play too.

King Josiah (the musical the guys did in fifth grade was based on this king) was a great example of a child who was obedient to God. When he was eight years old, he began his reign, a reign that included major reforms based on God's law. No one is ever too young to obey God. Read about it in II Kings 22:1-2. Psalm 8:2 reads: "From the lips of children and infants you have ordained praise." Children are often able to trust and praise God without doubts. Sometimes we have to become child-like again and remove barriers we have constructed so we can walk closer with God. There are no sabbaticals for us in our Christian life. We can't say, "Yeah, today I think I'll be a Christian but boy when that party comes up, I'm going to put my Christian life on hold." God wants us to live our "every square inch" for Him.

Thank you much for your prayers. I had an amazing weekend. I figured I'd be extremely tired on Saturday after staying out later on Friday night, but instead I was bursting with energy. I couldn't believe the bounce I had in my step, something I've been missing the past few months. I don't think I felt that good since before surgery. I'm convinced I had many prayer warriors lifting me up in prayer last week. Today we enjoyed a wonderful dinner at my parents' house, something we haven't done for a long time because I was usually too tired. I'm grateful to you and to God for this renewed strength. My feet feel almost completely normal and I can feel my fingers improving too. Oh, the blessings God sends! I'm forever grateful. My toenails and fingernails continue to loosen but I keep trimming them so I don't catch them on anything. It's a side effect I can live with.

Have a wonderful holiday and think of those of us at Dordt who will spend the day teaching.

Thursday, September 6, 2007 12:33 a.m.

Dear friends,

I've always been told that *Mr. Holland's Opus* was a good movie for educators to see, but I have never taken the time to watch it. Tonight I caught the last half hour of it. In that short time I didn't see what Glenn Holland did that was so impressive in the high school where he taught, but a comment that the governor of the state, an alumnus of the school, made at his farewell caught my attention. She said, "Look around you, Mr. Holland. There is not a life in this room that you have not touched.

And each one is a better person for meeting you or for being your student. This is your symphony, Mr. Holland. These people are the notes and melodies of your opus."

Each one of us is part of the symphony. We are the violins, the clarinets, the cellos that make up the composition. Each one of us adds our own beat, our own rhythm, our own notes. As we "make music," do we make the world a better place? Are the people around us better people because they have met us? As you work with people today, may you bless them with your song.

Psalm 103 is a great reminder to praise God with our whole being: "Praise the LORD, O my soul; all my inmost being, praise his holy name. . . . Praise the LORD, all his works everywhere in his dominion." Psalm 33:3 adds: "Sing to him a new song; play skillfully, and shout for joy." And Psalm 71:22, 23 reminds us: "I will praise you with the harp for your faithfulness, O my God; I will sing praise to you with the lyre, O Holy One of Israel. My lips will shout for joy when I sing praise to you— I, whom you have redeemed."

Make a joyful noise, today.

Friday, September 7, 2007 5:15 p.m.

Hello friends,

I don't usually write at this time of the week, but I wanted to share with you how well my week went. My students have been a blessing to me, as have my colleagues. It feels good to be back in class. My students energize me and have given me an incentive to get going each day. I'm very thankful for my job—for my students, my workplace, my coworkers. Today a couple of students stopped by to see how I was doing. My colleagues often offer to help and the secretary and work study have done much to help me. I'm grateful for all those around me who support me. I'm also very thankful for all of you who pray regularly for me. I have to add a thank you to Aunt Lucy who consistently sends me cards, even when she is struggling with her own health. God has blessed me with wonderful "seen and unseen" friends and I thank all of you.

Have a wonderful weekend, enjoying the beautiful fall weather. In Him.

Sunday, September 9, 2007 11:28 p.m.

Hello friends,

Last week I talked to my students in the Ed. Psych class to whom I teach the importance of building consistency into the young child's day.

When students know what to expect in their day, they build confidence and trust. Well, what is true for young children, I believe is true for adults too. Most people like a certain amount of consistency in their lives. That's what has been frustrating for me the past half year. Each time I think I have things figured out, things change.

Last weekend I had much energy and felt almost "normal" (whatever that means) once again. This weekend I was assuming it would be the same but as you may have guessed—it wasn't. I woke up feeling exhausted on Saturday morning. My body ached all over, from my toes (and I wore sensible shoes for three days) to my head. I struggled to get any work done but did manage to get some papers corrected. Late in the afternoon we went to Sioux Falls to attend a benefit for a friend of ours—Lorna Hunter. She was a nurse who helped us through many trying times when Josh was hospitalized in McKennan. We've stayed in touch over the years and even sat next to each other a few times in the infusion room. She wasn't able to attend the benefit because of many setbacks the past few months. She had pneumonia and a blood clot in her lung. Her cancer isn't growing but it isn't diminishing either. It was hard on me emotionally to hear of her struggles. My heart hurts for her and for her husband and two sons. Lorna's journey also reminds me that cancer is unpredictable and the unknown sometimes scares me. (She was cancer free for four and a half years after her first treatments.) And then I ran across one of my favorite verses—Isaiah 41:10: "So do not fear, for I am with you; do not be dismayed for I am your God. I will strengthen you and help you; I will uphold you with my righteous right hand." Once again I was comforted by God's Word. It reminded me that when I can't rely on being able to figure out what is going to happen, I know I can count on God to hold me and bring me the comfort I need for each day.

Thanks for your prayers and other ways you encourage me. Each day I thank God for all of you. Have a good week.

Wednesday, September 12, 2007 10:48 a.m.

Dear friends,

As I was saying last time, routines just don't seem to happen in my life. School was setting a nice routine for me. Even though I wasn't always sure about my sleep patterns, I could be pretty confident about my daily schedule. Classes, meetings, and advising have all pretty much followed as I thought and planned. Except, there always seem to be exceptions in my life. Josh has been bothered by his eye the past few days. Sunday he had a lot of pain and his vision seemed to be altered somewhat so I called my cousin Mick's office. Josh had planned to see him on Thursday, but with the new pain and vision problems, we thought we should call and tell him Josh's symptoms. Because Josh had a retina detachment shortly after his accident, the doctor (Mick was on his day off) said we should come in right away and have his eye looked at. So after my first class, I left with Joshua. Thankfully, a very competent ophthalmologist, after looking closely at his eye, determined that his present problems were not due to anything with his retina. He told us that his retina looks very good. We were thankful for that. He will see Dr. Mick on Thursday to see if they can determine what else is going on in his eye. Again, we are thankful for competent, kind, and caring doctors to whom we can look for help. We are also thankful for a kind, loving and caring Father who brings us through anxious moments.

Another reason to sing Psalm 56:3-4: "When I am afraid, I will trust in you. In God, whose word I praise, in God I trust; I will not be afraid."

Trusting in God for His care each day.

Thursday, September 13, 2007 7:14 a.m.

Dear friends,

It's a rainy morning here in Sanborn. After listening to the rain pitter-patter on our skylight, I was almost lulled into sleep again. But I'd had enough sleep for one day; last night's sleep actually equaled about two of my nights previously. I'm into another cyclical pattern—I'm tired so I lay down early, wake up because every inch of my body feels inflamed and is throbbing, get out the "traveling" ice pack, fall back to sleep, and wake up in the morning almost painless. I'm not quite sure why the pain hits me at about 12 o'clock but I know I'm very thankful for painkillers, anti-inflammatory medications, and the ice bag. I call it the "traveling" ice bag because I begin using it on my ankles and slowly move it up my body. The last place I use it is on my neck and in back of my head. It isn't real cold any more by that time so I can lay it directly on the sore areas. Isn't it wonderful to find remedies for our aches and pains?

Once again I am thankful for the encouragement I receive from you. After a day of teaching, I am usually pretty exhausted and often I come home to find something to cheer me up and keep me going. Often you remember Josh and Jerry too, and I'm thankful for that. Their part in all of this has involved their time and emotions too. Josh received a lovely note in one of our last cards and you could see how much it meant to him. Thank you! We have felt and continue to feel the love of our brothers and sisters in Christ. Our experience has shown us how to live out Romans 12:10: "Be devoted to one another in brotherly love."

Even without the shine from the sun, I hope you have a sun-shiny day.

Friday, September 14, 2007 6:41 a.m.

Hello friends,

Just to let you know, Josh went back to the ophthalmologist yesterday, this time to have his vision checked. My cousin Mick said Josh's eye is fine. He has 20/20 vision in both eyes, the inflammation is gone, and the tunnel vision has disappeared. We don't know what happened last weekend, but for now everything looks good. We are very thankful.

Yesterday I got to talk to Megan—until my phone card ran out. Megan sounded very upbeat: that always is good for a mother's heart! Amira is doing well at school and Nico is busy entertaining the guards and eating whenever he can. Mike's work is going very well; he's very happy with the progress.

I'm feeling much better today and getting ready for a wonderful day of teaching. I'm thankful for my job. My students and colleagues lift my spirits each day. I'm especially glad to be busy during the coming week. Even though I don't try to think about it, the upcoming PET scan weighs heavily on my mind. I trust that God will stand by me whatever the news, but the diagnosis, whatever it is, will again change my life. I hope you will continue to pray with me for the best news of all, that my lungs will once again be clear. That's the prayer I'm going to concentrate on right now. I'm going to travel through the coming week believing that God can cure, and that if the news is other than that, He'll give me what I need at that time. There is no sense borrowing trouble when it hasn't shown itself. I know my work will be a great diversion next week. As Matthew 6:34 tells us: "Therefore do not worry about tomorrow, for tomorrow will worry about itself. Each day has enough trouble of its own." The footnotes in my Bible said, "Planning for tomorrow is time well-spent, but worry is wasted time." Planning means setting goals and trusting in God's guidance. Worry, on the other hand, is being consumed by fear, which makes it difficult to trust God.

I pray each of you may have a wonderful day, enjoying those around you, encouraging those who you see need it. It's something you are good at. In Him.

Monday, September 17, 2007 12:00 a.m.

Hello dear friends,

Yesterday was a delightful day. My niece Emily (married to my nephew Michael) was baptized and made profession of faith. She grew up in the Apostolic Church which has the tradition of adult baptism so she had never been baptized. Because of her past traditions, she asked if she could be baptized by immersion rather than by sprinkling. So in the afternoon, we witnessed and celebrated her baptism at Lake Pahoja, a small lake near Inwood. It was a very touching ceremony. For me, personally, it was a visual reminder of the washing away of sin and the renewal of life in Jesus Christ.

After Emily's profession of faith, as the minister presented her with a devotional book, he read Psalm 37:3-6. I'm sure these verses meant much to Emily, but they also meant a lot to me, especially as I await my test this week. "Trust in the LORD and do good; dwell in the land and enjoy safe pasture. Delight yourself in the LORD and he will give you the desires of your heart. Commit your way to the LORD; trust in him and he will do this: He will make your righteousness shine like the dawn, the justice of your cause like the noonday sun." Verse 7 says, "Be still before the LORD and wait patiently for him. . . . " My Bible commentary said that committing my way to the Lord means entrusting everything to Him. Everything. It means I have to give my total trust to Him, believing that He will care for me better than I can care for myself. When I do this, I can "enjoy safe pasture." Enjoy the beautiful fall weather that's predicted for this week. In Him.

Tuesday, September 18, 2007 11:31 p.m.

Dear friends,

Trust, trust, trust! That's the gift that has been given to me over the past few days. I've been a little emotional this week, but surprisingly calm. I feel a complete trust in God. I didn't get that on my own. I thank God for the miraculous way He has worked in my life. (You can probably say the same.) Today in the chapel service I attended, I was reminded of the importance of trusting in God. My colleagues reminded me to trust and so did many of you. I, of course, have some apprehensions as Thursday approaches, but I do trust that God will provide for my physical and emotional needs no matter what news I receive. Isaiah 12:2 says, "Surely God is my salvation; I will trust and not be afraid."

I have an extremely busy day tomorrow. I have individual conferences with the sixteen freshmen who are in my Gen 100 class. That should keep my mind occupied. Thanks for all your support.

Wednesday, September 19, 2007 11:58 p.m.

To all my dear friends,

Barbara Johnson, best-selling author and comedienne, tells a story about a little boy. It could be a story about any of my grandchildren because they all love to climb into their parents' bed, frightened or not frightened. One night a little boy, frightened by the sound of the wind, toddled off to find his parents, waking his father with his sobs. The father walked his son back to his bedroom and promised he would lie with him until he fell asleep again. As they were lying in the darkness, the little boy whispered, "Daddy, I can't see you. Are you still here?"

"Yes, son I'm here," the father answered. Not quite sure, the boy said, "I can't see you, Daddy. Is your face turned toward me?" "Yes son, my face is turned toward you."

That's what I want to know tomorrow as I lie quietly on the table, waiting for the radioactive dye to spread through my body, as my body travels in and out of the tunnel, and as I receive the report and Dr. Krie's recommendation for treatment. Are You here God? Can You see me? Is Your face still turned toward me? And I'm sure the answer will be the same as it has been my whole life: always.

Many of you have reminded me of God's faithfulness and the importance of trusting Him, whatever the report may be. He is able to heal and He is also able to comfort. I pray that my response tomorrow will reveal my trust in God. "Blessed is the man who fears the LORD . . . . He will have no fear of bad news; his heart is steadfast, trusting in the LORD" (Psalm 112:1,7). I've shed a few tears the past few days, but most of them haven't been tears of sadness. The tears I've shed have been because so many of you have touched my life in a tremendous way, encouraging me to believe in God's power.

Thank you for everything. In Him.

Thursday, September 20, 2007 3:27 p.m.

Just a quick note to let you all know that we are praising God for the wonderful news we received today. The PET scan showed no cancer in my lungs. We are thanking God for His power in healing and granting it to me. I'll write more later.

THANKS FOR ALL YOUR PRAYERS! In Him.

Friday, September 21, 2007 12:07 a.m.

Up, down, all around, upside down and inside out. That kind of describes my emotions yesterday. One minute I was sure the cancer was gone and the next I was worried that my cough or the pain in my chest meant the return of cancer. Anxiety built as we rode to Sioux Falls early Thursday morning. I wanted the scan to be over so I knew what I had to deal with. It took about two hours to complete the scan. I was thankful that I hadn't slept well Wednesday night so I could sleep through most of it. Later as I walked out the door of the clinic holding the white envelope with the film inside, I wondered what news it held. I wondered what path my life would take. Oh how I wanted to peek; but I knew it was sealed for a purpose. I had to wait for Dr. Krie to read the scan.

We spent the next couple of hours shopping but it was the cheapest shopping trip Jerry ever took me on. I couldn't concentrate on anything. I kept focusing on the faces of the technicians as I left their office. It seemed to me they were very somber—did that mean they had detected something on the scan? So many thoughts ran through my head. Finally it was time to meet with Dr. Krie. I had my blood drawn and then waited to be called into Dr. Krie's office. As Dr. Krie walked into the room where we were waiting, she quickly began asking me about the pain in my joints I had told Kathy (the nurse) about. I was wondering, "When is she going to tell me the results?" At the same time I was glad for the diversion because I was afraid of what I might hear. After asking some questions, she finally said, "Well, do you want to hear the good news?" We picked up on her word "good" immediately. She went on to explain that the scan had showed absolutely no cancer. The nodules were gone. Everything was clear. It's hard to explain how we responded. Even though we had prayed hard for this and we knew many people had been praying for the very thing that Dr. Krie was telling us, we could hardly believe it. We were so happy and excited that we could hardly respond.

Finally, after asking Dr. Krie if she was really sure, we couldn't stop asking questions. Now what? What if? Will it stay away? What's going to happen now? After some discussion, Dr. Krie suggested I take Xeloda, a chemo that comes in pill form, as a precaution. She wanted to make sure that we understood that although the cancer is gone for now, there is always the chance that it will return at some point because it had metastasized. We understand that, but for now, we will take the good news and pray that the cancer will continue to stay in remission. The days ahead will still have their trials. The new drug comes with its own set of side effects, one being hand-and-foot syndrome. I have to begin immediately to take very good care of my hands and feet to avoid blisters, rash, and broken skin. But we're not going to borrow trouble before it is here, and we are going to thank God for each new day. Each day is a day to be celebrated. As the Psalmist says in Psalm 118, "This is the day that the LORD has made; let us rejoice and be glad in it . . . . You are my God, and I will give you thanks; you are my God, and I will exalt you" (vs. 24, 29).

God always hears and answers our prayers. This time He answered, "Yes." I'm sure Jerry and I don't have any idea how many prayers were offered on our behalf. Even though we would like to, we can't begin to say thanks to each of you in person, but please know that we appreciate and thank you for every prayer that you have uttered. We hope that you will now help us thank Him. "Give thanks to the LORD, for he is good; his love endures forever" (vs. 30). In Him.

Tuesday, September 25, 2007 12:49 a.m.

Dear friends,

The weekend was a busy one. My good news seemed to give me renewed energy. Catherine and I took Chyann and the boys to the Dordt Pops Concert on Friday night. On Saturday I cleaned out my flower beds, getting them ready for winter and hosted a kick-off for our Bible study group. On Sunday we took an afternoon road trip around O'Brien county with dear friends from Luverne and Sanborn.

Throughout the whole weekend I was physically busy, but my mind was also busy—busy thinking about a question that continues to plague me, something I haven't been able to get out of my mind. What now? What am I to learn from this experience? Although I am very grateful, I ask, "Why, God, have you healed me?" I don't want to take away from the beauty of the healing and the gratitude I feel, but yet this burdens me. It's the same questions I've had when I returned from Nigeria. All these experiences give me the feeling that I should do something with them, but what? Is there something different, or more, or bigger, or is it just a reminder to stay faithful to God, faithful in my actions, faithful in my relationships, faithful as a wife and mother, faithful as a teacher, faithful as a church member, faithful in my community, faithful in my use of resources, faithful in my finances. Sometimes big experiences change us, but I think in the realm of life, they are best used as a reminder to be faithful in all that God has given us. What does faithful mean? What does faithful look like? Being faithful isn't generic; it isn't a recipe that you can follow. Being faithful is going to mean something different and look different to different people. Faithfulness is an important quality. It involves action as well as attitudes. Our lives reveal if we are truly faithful.

Proverbs 3:3 reads: "Let love and faithfulness never leave you; bind them around your neck, write them on the tablet of your heart." God has given us a great model of faithfulness. Psalm 117: 2b reads: " . . . The faithfulness of the LORD endures forever." We continue to see this in our lives.

I started on my new chemo pills yesterday. It is surely much more convenient than driving to an infusion center. I'll take these pills for two weeks, wait a week, then see Dr. Krie who will check my blood and check for side effects. In the meantime, I hope to continue to enjoy teaching, being a grandma, mother, and wife, playing for church services, and enjoying the beautiful people God has placed beside me, trying to be faithful in all that I do. In Him.

Wednesday, September 26, 2007 11:36 p.m.

Dear friends,

As you may have noticed from a few of the entries, today is my birthday. When you are a teacher, birthdays are always fun. Students love to celebrate with you, even in college. But to be honest, I haven't looked forward to my birthdays the last few years. It meant that I got older. But this year it was different. I am very glad to be one year older. Isn't it amazing how a perspective can change? I feel a new appreciation for life, a joy in being able to celebrate being another year older. I wonder if this feeling I have is a little like David's when he said in Psalm 30:11-12: "You turned my wailing into dancing; you removed my sackcloth and clothed me with joy, that my heart may sing to you and not be silent. O LORD, my God, I will give you thanks forever." I give thanks to God today for giving me reason to dance and sing. I pray I will continue to thank Him forever. I hope you too find things to dance and sing about.

Thanks for the birthday wishes. I love being another year older!

Wednesday, October 31, 2007 3:39 a.m.

To my Dear friends,

I can't believe it has been this long since I've written in my journal. I've missed you. You probably have gotten the picture that school has kept me busy! I'm thankful that I am teaching this semester. My work, my colleagues, and my students have been an inspiration. Preparing lectures, dreaming up creative ways to get information to students, correcting student work, meeting with students, writing letters of recommendation, and attending meetings makes my days fly. The extreme fatigue that

I felt while on the infused chemo is gone. I do get tired after a day's work but it isn't that intense tiredness. It's sort of like old times—tiredness because of too little sleep.

A bit more about what's been happening:

About five weeks ago I began taking an oral chemo. It's really easy; I just pop pills into my mouth each morning and evening. Even though that sounds easy, it is a bit difficult for me, for you see, I really detest taking pills. But each time I think about complaining, I tell myself how much better this is than going in for an infusion. The oral pill Xeloda has worked well for me in many ways. One side effect of the medication is hand-and-foot syndrome which I soon found out about. The first dose went well (I take the pills for two weeks and then have one week off). After I began the second round, I began to notice some pain in my feet. My fingers are still affected by the neuropathy that developed from the first medication but they haven't been "hit" by the second side effect. I limped around for a few days, gave up my fun shoes, and finally called Dr. Krie. She suggested I stop the medication a few days early, take my week off and then develop our next plan. So I've been sitting while I teach, wearing flip-flops (they are the only shoes I can stand on my feet), applying all kinds of lotions to my feet, and enjoying time off from popping pills. I'll see Dr. Krie on Friday when she will probably put me on a lower dose of Xeloda which I hope will prevent my feet from feeling as if I'm walking on nails.

Since I've written last, I've come into contact with many people who suffer from illnesses, depression, anxiety, and other conflicts. It's such a reminder of all the brokenness that we suffer from in this world. And yet, among the brokenness, we have the assurance that our great, big, beautiful God is in control. Among the brokenness, we can see how He is always present and always working.

Mar, the verses you suggested in Psalm 16 and Acts 2 were great. As we think about God's constant presence, we find contentment. The footnote talks about the difference between happiness and joy. Happiness comes and goes and is based on external circumstances but joy is lasting and is based on God's presence within us. When we face the future, whether it looks scary or filled with doubt or uncertainty, we can be confident that God will be there with us, knowing our needs even before we do. What a reminder: we must base our future on God.

Psalm 16:8-11 reads: "I have set the LORD always before me. Because he is at my right hand, I will not be shaken. Therefore my heart is glad and my tongue rejoices; my body also will rest secure, because you will not abandon me to the grave, nor will you let your Holy One see decay. You made known to me the path of life; you will fill me with joy in your presence, with eternal pleasures at your right hand."

Thanks for your continued prayers and thoughtful ways. I received a month-late birthday card today which reminded me that every day is a day to be celebrated! Being specific, you can pray for relief from pain in my fingers and feet so that I can go back on my chemo pills in a few days. I continue to thank God for you, for being able to teach, for modern medicine, and people who develop and administer treatments.

I hope you are enjoying the wonderful fall weather as much as I am. I love you all!

P.S. If you are checking the time I wrote this journal, you're probably wondering what I'm doing up at this time of the morning. I woke up a little bit ago because of pain in my feet so I got out my pop cans and started rolling them back and forth. Modern medicine is wonderful, but simple things can be effective too.

Saturday, November 3, 2007 12:50 a.m.
Hello friends,

It's been a long week—lots of meetings, lectures that were hard to prepare for, and students with problems. Although I'm tired I am very glad for work that is satisfying and rewarding. Dr. Krie was in Sioux Center today so I slipped out of the office for a short time this morning for a checkup. A checkup always involves having my blood tested. Each time I wait for the results, I feel a little anxious about what I will hear. But once again, the results were wonderful. My counts continue to stay in the normal range. Each time I thank God for His wonderful care. Because my feet continue to pain me (Dr. Krie said I have broken blood vessels in the pads of my feet), I won't be able to continue chemo for another week. I hope I'll be able to begin taking the oral treatments again on the 12th of November. She suggested I take vitamin B6; have any of you heard of this helping hand-and-foot syndrome? She suggested I stay off my feet as much as possible. After my appointment, I went back to campus to teach a class and thought I would try to heed her suggestion. So as I began to lecture, I decided it would be a good idea to climb onto the new high chair they have provided in the classroom. Not as easy done as said. This nice new stool is high, doesn't have arms to help you balance, and the seat twists. So there I was trying to climb on it as it was turning and twisting and slipping away from me. What I'd like to have done is to climb on the table and then plop myself in the chair but that wouldn't have looked too sophisticated, but then again neither did trying to hop on it from the floor. Anyway, after a few tries, I did land on the seat. That was probably the closest I've come to having all my students' attention this semester. But sitting on the stool only lasted a short time. It's really hard for me to teach from a sitting position. After about five minutes I said to my students, "I've got two weeks before Dr. Krie is going to check my feet again, so I'm going to forget the chair for today and try again next week." I'll continue to swab my feet with lotion, roll them on cold pop cans, and keep them up as much as possible. I was told in no uncertain terms that I must wear comfortable shoes so I guess I'll pack the high heels away for awhile. Flip-flops have worked well this week, but the cold temperatures that are predicted for next week could pose problems.

This week I decided to stop wearing my hats. Although my hair is very short, at least it covers my head and the bald spots have filled in. My hair is much greyer than I remember it before treatments, but at this point I don't care. It's just nice to have hair again after one half year. One thing I've learned through this experience is to be content with my circumstances. I thought it would be more difficult to lose my hair (although I did find it very difficult to lose my eyelashes and my eyebrows). It is amazing how things that once seemed important have taken a back seat when you're fighting to get rid of cancer. I was okay with losing my hair, if it meant the disease could be treated. And now I'm okay with having really short hair. God has a great way of helping us put things in perspective. My students, colleagues, family and friends have been tremendously supportive and encouraging which, of course, makes everything easier.

I continually thank God for all of you, for your prayers, for your support, for your encouragement. In Him.

Sunday, November 4, 2007 10:42 p.m.
Dear friends,

My Gen. 100 class came over for dinner today. It was great to have them in our home and see them outside the school setting. I'm always thankful for Jerry, but on days like today I especially appreciate him. He is a great helper in the kitchen and a superb griller.

The down side is that I discovered that the more I work with my hands, the more painful they get. It isn't really my hands, it's my fingers. I used to think the pain was left over from the neuropathy caused from the Paxil and Avastin, but after using my hands to open cans, mix up pudding and Cool Whip, stir the chocolate and peanut butter, I'm wondering if I'm not feeling the hand-and-foot syndrome in my hands too. Since I sat down to do much of the preparing, my feet actually feel pretty good, but my fingers itch and tingle. On top of cooking, I also practiced the piano and organ for the morning service on Sunday, which probably added to the discomfort. With hand-and-foot syndrome, discomfort comes from putting pressure on the affected areas. That's why standing and walking hurt my feet and carrying objects and grasping things tightly hurt my fingers. Discomfort comes from the pressure.

Sometimes we feel pressure in life too. We get the squeeze put on us and we feel uncomfortable. Sometimes that squeeze comes from choices that we make—choices that break the norms that were established by God in His act of creation. Sometimes we recognize our errant ways when we read His Word and we see how inadequately we live up to it. But thankfully, just as changing my behavior (with my hands and feet) changes the pain in my fingers and toes, the squeeze can be lessened when I change my behavior in life too. Sitting on high chairs (see last entry), rolling my feet on pop cans, asking others to open bottles and cans won't work to alleviate sin, but reading God's Word and applying it to my life will. As it is very important right now that I "follow the rules" to rid my feet and hands from pain, it is just as important that I follow God's Word to help me stay away from sin. Following His Word doesn't mean I won't have pain in my life, but it will help me fight the sin that is ready to show up in my life. Some days I struggle with taking the time to read God's Word, and yet every day that I do, I am blessed by His reminders, His comfort, His assurance, His rules for faithful living, and much more.

In my Gen. 100 class, we are talking about developing habits that will improve our Christian walk. One of the habits they have chosen to work on is the habit of developing their devotional life. For the next two weeks they are committing themselves to reading the Bible and journaling. For some of my students it means they will work on deepening a habit they have already established. For others, it is finding a regular time and a quiet space to read and study the Bible. For me, I'm committing myself to a deeper study of God's Word too. If you take time to spend time with God, good for you. If not, try taking time to read about God from His Word.

Psalm 119 has many wonderful verses that talk about reading God's Word. Verses 97 and 105 say, "Oh, how I love your law! I meditate on it all day long . . . . Your word is a lamp to my feet and a light for my path."

Have a good week.

Thursday, November 8, 2007 12:28 a.m.

Dear friends,

Tonight I was in the B.J. Haan Auditorium at Dordt with almost the entire Dordt freshman class plus other Dordt students, professors, and community people. We were there to listen to Tony Campolo, a sociologist who was invited to Dordt as part of an annual lecture series. If you've ever heard Dr. Campolo, you know that we were challenged. Through his funny stories and dynamic presentation, we were emphatically and passionately challenged to live a life that shows that Jesus is the Lord of our life. He told us about a time in his life when he believed that Jesus came to earth to bring him to the next life, but as he grew in wisdom, he came to understand that Jesus came to invade our lives and transform us so that we can become agents of change in a world that is very much influenced by Satan but controlled by God. He challenged the students to work hard to receive a good education but to use it—not to climb the social ladder of success, buying into our North American culture where a good education leads to a good job which leads to making a lot of money which allows for us to buy a lot of stuff—but to be transformers of society.

Campolo told the story of friend of his, a Harvard lawyer, who could have made thousands of dollars by taking a corporate job but instead chose to work in the prison system in Montgomery, Alabama, where he works to defend the prisoners on death row. He reminded us that many of the people on death row are the poor, those who don't have the money to hire a good lawyer. This lawyer is good and in his work at transforming a system, he is transforming lives. That's what God calls us to do. As Campolo said, God calls us to love the unlovable. Christ said it is easy to love those who are like us, those we can easily love, but we are called to reach out to those who might disgust us or make us squirm or make us feel uncomfortable. Campolo told the story about the derelict he met on a "skid row" street. The man wanted to give him a hug because he was feeling so blessed (he'd been given a cup of coffee). Campolo wasn't too excited about getting that close to the smelly man. But as the man hugged him, he remembered the verse from Matthew 25 which talks about the hungry, the thirsty, the homeless, the stranger, the sick, and the prisoner. At the end of chapter 25, Jesus reminds us that there will be those who ask, "Lord, when did we see you hungry or thirsty or a stranger or needing clothes or sick or in prison, and did not help you?" Jesus replies: "I tell you the truth, whatever you did not do for one of the least of these, you did not do for me."

We (at least I) continue to need to be reminded to seek out the poor and in some small way change a life, one person, one situation at a time. God has blessed us both materially and spiritually. What are we willing to do to show that He is Lord of our life?

My hands and feet continue to be a source of concern. Tonight I stood too long and immediately my feet turned red, began to itch, and started to hurt. I really notice immediately when I put pressure on my hands and feet. My hands are beginning to heal from putting too much pressure on them last weekend. This syndrome is really crazy. A few days after I've been too hard on my hands or feet, the skin begins to peel. I'm hoping to begin treatment again on Monday, so I have to be careful. For this round, the dosage will be cut down by about one-third in the hope that I will be able to tolerate it better.

Again, we are thankful for the ways you continue to remember us. I'm grateful for the cards, words of encouragement, and the prayers with which you continue to bless us. We are amazed and humbled that you continue to think of us. It's that cold cup of water.

Tuesday, November 13, 2007 12:55 a.m.

Hello friends,

I want to give you a quick update on what is happening with my treatments.

Today I began my chemo pills again. Dr. Krie set this date to try it again, only this time with a lesser dose. So this morning and this evening, I once again took the pills but this time I took only four instead of six. I plan to be very careful with my feet. I'll wear only sensible shoes and walk and stand as little as possible. I hope this will keep my feet from becoming irritated, red, swollen and sore. As I said earlier, it is very difficult to teach without standing, but I'll have to try. I've been wearing shoes instead of flip-flops for the past week so we'll see if that continues to work.

I had my port flushed today. Now that I am not having infusions, I have to have saline and heparin pushed through my port about once a month to keep it functional. It takes only a minute to have the solutions injected but the sanitation process takes much longer. They are very careful not to cause an infection.

Over the past few weeks, I've been reminded over and over again of all the prayers that have/are being offered on my behalf. I feel blessed to have so many people who are willing to continue to pray. Thanks much! At this time you can pray that I can ward off the hand-and-foot syndrome and continue with the chemo. The application of this chemo is two weeks on and one week off and then back on again. Dr. Krie says she hopes we can keep this up for about a year. We'll have to see how it goes. I will be having another PET scan right after the first of the year.

I'm very grateful for all of you!

Tuesday, November 13, 2007 11:20 p.m.

Dear friends,

Last night I was part of a panel that discussed the Tony Campolo lectures. The group consisted of mostly upperclassmen and a few professors. It was interesting to hear how differently people interpreted the message Campolo presented. Even though what Campolo said held different meaning for various members of the audience, there was one theme that seemed to come through loud and clear: God calls each of us to extend His kingdom each and every day. One question that Campolo said he asks himself each morning is, "What can I do today to fulfill God's kingdom?" At night he asks himself, "What did I do today to enhance God's kingdom?" Those are good questions for each of us to ask ourselves. It seems (at least for me) that it is easy to live for my own enjoyment or my own satisfaction, and when a busy day has ended, I'm too tired even to ask the question. Being reflective is something that makes me conscious of where I am and what I am doing. Tony's main theme is making a difference for those who are oppressed. Last night it was obvious that we are not doing enough to change the world. We discussed some of the big things that have to change in our society like (just to name a few things) an over-emphasis on materialism and entertainment. Many things were suggested but often the suggestions seem to run into roadblocks. It isn't easy to come up with a solution. Part of the reason is that we are all (Christians included) so caught up in our culture that we really don't want to change. We don't want to be counter-cultural. In fact, we kind of like the advantages we have. But as we talked, one thing became evident: we can make big changes only if we are first willing to make small changes in our life. This includes being stewardly with the resources that we have, being conscious of the way we care for God's world, living simply—(how many pairs of shoes can one have)? We must learn about what is going on in the world and share what we know with others, stand up for those around us who are marginalized, take a look at our own lives, and be open to see where we can change. There are many ways in which we can make a difference if we are willing to step outside our own little boxes and take risks.

Proverbs 14:31 says: "He who oppresses the poor shows contempt for their Maker, but whoever is kind to the needy honors God."

The chemo pills seem to have hit my stomach hard this time. I feel hungry but when I eat, I feel miserable. I think I'll have to be more careful what I eat when I take my pills. I just read that the pills should always be taken with water, which I haven't always been doing. So I'll change that and see if that helps. I was exhausted today, something I haven't experienced for about two weeks. I'm hoping that as my body gets accustomed to the pills, I'll tolerate them better. My hands feel much better today. I always have a certain amount of pain after I play piano for a church service, which I did on Sunday. It takes a pretty strong strike on the keys to play for congregational singing and that usually leads to pain. The good thing is that the pain usually subsides after a few days. And I love playing so much that I'm willing to suffer through a little pain. Someone asked if typing (which I do a lot of) did the same thing, but it doesn't. I strike the piano keys with the tips of my fingers and the keyboard with the bottom of my fingers. Interesting, huh? Tomorrow is another rousing day so I think I'll get ready for it by going to bed and getting a good night's sleep.

I continue to love to hear from you! I hope that each of you has a day full of joy and that as you enjoy your day, you look for ways that you can help the world become a place filled with shalom. In Him.

Monday, November 19, 2007 8:34 p.m.

Hello friends,

On again, off again. That's the best way I can describe my chemo treatments. After about ten days of being off my chemo treatments and then seven days on, I went in to Dr. Krie today to see if I could continue and take the next seven days of pills. The decision was going to be based on my feet. All I was supposed to do today was run in, lift my feet, and go back to work. Since my feet have been feeling fine, I didn't anticipate it being any big deal. Over the past three weeks, I've been very careful not to stand for too long and I've only worn sensible shoes. Every once in a while I'll slip on a pair of pretty, tall high heels, but only for a minute. Before I left this morning, I followed my routine of swabbing my feet with lotion. Immediately I noticed some broken blisters which I flicked at and soon discovered that I could peel off almost all the skin from the bottom of my right foot. It came off in big chunks. Not good. When I tipped my foot to take a look, it was bright red. Even though I didn't feel pain, I was afraid of Dr. Krie's diagnosis. Sure enough, I popped into the office for a quick show of my feet, and she decided that I couldn't afford to let my feet get worse. We sat for a while and discussed what she hoped for in the future and what kind of plan I would follow. This is what she decided—I'll stay off my pills for the next seven days and if my feet get better, I'll go back on for seven days. I'll stay at the lower dose (2000 mg) for now but she would like to increase the dosage soon. I'll keep up the seven days on, seven days off cycle for as long as I can tolerate the medication. Dr. Krie has had one patient on the medication for two years. She said the one week on, one week off rotation has proven to be as effective as the two weeks on, one week off. So we'll see how it goes.

Later today, when I had time to think about it, I reflected on today's change of plans and all the changes that have happened in my life over the past months. One of the things that struck me is being able to take things as they come. I haven't always been like that. I could worry, fret, wish for better reports, dwell on the negative, but none of those things is going to change what has or is to happen. I've learned to trust that alternative plans are okay. I've learned a new meaning to: "Trust in the LORD with all your heart and lean not on your own understanding; in all your ways acknowledge him and he will make your paths straight," and "Be joyful in hope, patient in affliction, and faithful in prayer" (Romans 12:12).

I don't know what my path is going to look like in the future but I do know that the only way I'll be able to handle the curves, the road-blocks, and the sharp turns is to turn to Jesus and let Him take hold and take care of me. I've seen His care shown in many ways—just recently I received a beautiful box of "feet" things from my cousin Mick and his wife Judy. I'm hoping the wonderful bath salts will help soften and soothe my feet. The special socks are comfortable and keep the lotion on my feet as I sleep at night.

Thanksgiving is coming and I have much to be thankful for. I'm thankful for all my friends (old and new). I continue to be thankful and humbled by all the prayers you've offered on my behalf. Last Sunday, Laura, a friend from the past whom I haven't seen for years, reminded me that she continues to pray for me daily. Just another reminder of God's faithfulness being shown through His people. I'm thankful for advice, encouragement, funny jokes and stories that you've shared, and unexpected "boxes." Have a good week!

Thursday, November 22, 2007 12:43 a.m.

Hello my dear friends,

Yesterday I spent much of the day sitting in my comfy chair with my feet up, grading papers, previewing videos for a class, and looking at materials for next week. I've also spent some time thinking about today, a day we've set aside for giving specific thanks for all the blessings we've experienced over the past year.

Today I'm thankful for the comforts of my home. I think of those who lack these comforts. I'm thankful for friends and family. I think of those who have strained relationships. I'm thankful for people who encourage, support, and pray. I'm also thankful for surprise packages, cards, and words of encouragement. I think of those who are forgotten. I'm thankful for wonderful medical services, facilities, and medicines, even when they have side effects. I'm sorry for those who don't have this opportunity. I'm thankful for e-mail and calling cards so that we can "talk" to our family in Abuja, Nigeria. I'm sorry for those who can't or don't desire to keep contact. I'm very thankful for all my grandchildren (Kobi, Amira, Bailey, Nico, and Miles). I hope everyone gets to experience this joy in their life. I'm thankful for books and music and flowers and all the lovely things that bring joy.

Thanksgiving has a new meaning for me this year. I'm thankful for big things in life, but I'm also thankful for the little things that last year at this time I didn't even think about, like hair that blows in the wind. Yes, I felt mine blow last week! At first I wasn't sure, but after standing still for a bit I'm sure it really happened. Would you believe, I'm even thankful for grey hair? (And I'm thankful for hairdressers (Stacy) who can take care of that.) I'm thankful for hats that covered my head when I lost my hair. I'm thankful for feet and hands, even if they are peeling. I'm thankful for low, comfy shoes, even if they don't make me look taller and slimmer. I'm thankful for lotions, many that were given to me by you. I'm thankful for needing only normal hours of sleep after having to sleep for many hours a few months ago. I'm thankful for chemo pills which I can take when it is convenient. And the list could go on and on.

I'm really thankful for great friends and family who have stood beside us through this whole journey. I'm tremendously thankful for students, colleagues, and a workplace that has supported me the whole way. I'm thankful for a church family that encouraged us in many ways. I'm especially thankful to God who has heard our prayers, yours and mine, and has sent healing. I don't know what tomorrow will bring, but after once again seeing God's faithfulness day after day, I know I can count on Him never letting go.

I Thessalonians 5:16-18 reads: "Be joyful always; pray continually; give thanks in all circumstances, for this is God's will for you in Christ Jesus." Paul didn't say give thanks for all things; he said to give thanks in all things. When bad things happen we don't necessarily thank Him for them, but we thank Him for His presence and for the good He can do through the circumstance.

I hope you all take time to think of all of the ways God has blessed you this year, from the big to the little. Your thanks will look different than mine, but I imagine you will find plenty of blessings for which to thank God—blessings for an enjoyable, refreshing, thankful day.

Saturday, November 24, 2007 11:58 p.m.

A new look! My appearance has changed quite a bit the last three-quarters of a year, not that I planned for it to change. In case you didn't catch it from earlier journal entries, just recently I've ditched my hats for my real, very short, very grey hair. I'm used to it now, but when I unexpectedly catch a glimpse of myself in a mirror, I'm still surprised at how I look. It still doesn't look like me. I haven't had my hair short since I was a freshman in high school, and even then it wasn't this short. I forget about my new "look" until I meet someone who hasn't seen me in a while, and they remind me of it with either a quizzical look or something they say.

I changed the look of my site too. It matches the seasons; well maybe not yet, but the forecasters say our weather will be changing. The cold has already set in; snow is coming.

Change is good. Michael and Megan are finding out that even though they love warm weather, they do miss the change of the seasons. Change not only makes our life more interesting but it can be good for us too. It is something that can make us ponder and reflect, stretch and search, evaluate and consider. A guest minister we had many years back mentioned that if we weren't changing, we were actually going backwards. He said that staying the same is not really staying the same at all. If we aren't moving forward, we're going backward. He didn't believe we could stay the same. Interesting perspective, huh? As Christians we constantly have to be evaluating our lives. We know that God's Word is static. It doesn't change, but our understanding of it does. As we struggle with the text, as we reflect on how it changes our lives, we gain wisdom. We see that God's Word in our life should be dynamic. Our lives should be ever changing as we grow and experience life. As Malachi 3:6 says, "I, the LORD do not change." It's an interesting chapter; I hope you take time to read it sometime.

Just as we can be guaranteed that the weather is going to change, we can be sure that life will change. Sometimes we don't like the change, but we can be sure that if we see how God works through it and uses it to help us search for Him more and more, our lives are enriched. I'm not looking forward to winter, and yet I know it will be another season of growth. Sort of like life, right? Have a wonderful Sunday.

Monday, November 26, 2007 1:22 a.m.

Good Day,

I know that I've commented on Psalm 92 previously, but through the sermon I listened to Sunday, I was again reminded of the beauty of this Psalm. It begins by telling us that it is good to praise the Lord. The NIV commentary reminded me that it is important to give thanks to God for His abundant blessings, not only during the Thanksgiving holiday, but praise should be on our lips every day. There are many things for which we can be thankful: family, friends, church, leaders, material things—all things that come to us from God. The commentary stated that when we become thankful, our attitude in life changes. It said we will become more "positive, gracious, loving and humble." Think of people who are content and you will recognize these characteristics in them. The psalmist goes on to say that the righteous will flourish like a palm tree. H-m-m a palm tree! I've always loved palm trees. They are unique and something so different from the trees I've seen all my life. They stand tall and erect, always looking to the heavens. What makes a palm tree unique to the psalmist? Palm trees are known for their long life. They are known for putting more energy into their fruit than the tree. They are known to resist being grafted. The palm tree can produce fruit even in a dry climate. The palm tree has long roots that go deep.

How does this compare with a Christian's life? We too should look different from the world around us. We should be known for our love for God and for our desire to live a life that holds to His commandments. We should be putting more energy into what we produce (fruits of the spirit, etc.) than what we look like and what we possess. We should resist the culture around us that wants us to buy into materialism, individualism, to over-emphasize recreation and other cultural desires. Last night our minister said that a palm tree, unlike other trees, will not grow around an object. That was interesting to me. Last year our son-in-law Mike showed us a deciduous tree in their backyard that had grown along a fence. As it was growing it got "caught" in the fence and for a short while grew sideways, following the fence until it came to a supporting pole which it followed up until it ran out of metal. The palm tree wouldn't do this; it wouldn't have grafted itself into the fence. It would have continued to grow straight. Like the palm tree, we too must have roots that grow deep. Those roots grow deep by being in constant contact with God's Word.

That brings us back to the first two verses where the psalmist begins by saying, "It is good to praise the LORD and make music to your name, O Most High, to proclaim your love in the morning and your faithfulness at night" (vs. 1-2). The psalmist knows that our source of life is found in our relationship with God. That is why it is good to praise the Lord. It is through worship that we commune with God. The introduction to the Psalm indicates that it is a song for the Sabbath day. On the Sabbath day, our faith is renewed and our life restored as our roots grow deep as we commune with God. The psalmist says that the result will be a life that flourishes like a palm tree; a tree that bears fruit, even in old age.

A quick update: My feet are still peeling. My right foot has fresh new skin over the entire bottom while my left foot has more skin to shed. I've lost a bit of skin off the tips of my fingers, but it is only minimal. My feet actually hurt much less than they did a few weeks ago. The new skin is tender and, of course, there's a little pain where I tore the skin that wasn't quite ready to come off. My cousin Mar Sjaarda gave me some new lotion this weekend so my feet have yet another source of hydration. Thanks, Mar.

Tomorrow morning I'm going to see a rheumatoidologist. Dr. Krie made the appointment with this doctor about two months ago when I was having a lot of pain in my joints. The pain has really decreased so I was tempted to cancel it, but since I've struggled with joint pain for many years, I decided it is probably a good idea to have a good checkup by a specialist. Who knows, maybe she'll have a good remedy for my hip pain. I'll also be reporting to Dr. Krie to see if I can begin my chemo pills today. I'm hoping she'll let me begin again.

I hope you all have a great week. I also hope that as you work and play, others will recognize you as a palm tree. In Him.

Tuesday, November 27, 2007 1:51 a.m.

The rheumatoidologist confirmed what I suspected—she is quite sure my pain isn't coming from rheumatoid arthritis. She ordered blood tests (I don't think I've ever filled up so many little vials) and x-rays which she will discuss with me over Christmas vacation. For now she put me on some medication that we hope will relieve the pain in my joints. I talked for a while with Dr. Krie this morning and she decided I could go back on Xeloda, the chemo pill. I'll take a smaller dose for a while and see how my hands and feet handle it. Right now both my hands and feet feel pretty good. I keep swabbing on the lotion. Last night my hands were hurting, so I covered them with lotion and then (because I was too lazy to go look for gloves) I put socks over them. Looked a little ridiculous but felt good!

Even though I've been very grateful for the two good reports I had today, my heart is heavy with recent news from friends. One friend was just diagnosed with breast cancer and I'm waiting to hear her prognosis. Another friend, from the days our daughters were in Western, was involved in an accident in which her daughter was killed. At this time of year, when we've just spent time in thanksgiving and look forward to the joy of Christmas, there seems little thanks and little joy in the life of my two friends. They are both hurting. Both must have fears and questions. As I thought about my friends' circumstances I was reminded again of the verses that I spoke of last week. "Be joyful always; pray continually; give thanks in all circumstances" (I Thessalonians 5:16-18). I can't imagine anyone giving thanks for these circumstances but knowing my two friends, I'm sure they are giving thanks that in their circumstances God is present in their lives. He is there, holding them, comforting them and bringing people into their lives to stand by their sides. I hope you will join me in praying that they will find peace during this hurting time. Thanks.

Thursday, November 29, 2007 6:51 a.m.

Hello dear friends,

When I woke up this morning it took me awhile to think about my feet. That's a good thing. That means I wasn't feeling any pain or discomfort. It's been a while since that happened. When I did think about my feet, I stretched them, flipped them back and forth and then thought, "Sure enough, they are there, but they don't hurt." My next thought was, "Thank you, God!" Through all of this—this journey of cancer and surgery, chemo and side effects—God has patiently been there, sometimes walking beside me, sometimes carrying me, but always there. During this time, I've read scripture, heard sermons, studied devotionals, sought out wise people, all the time learning more about God. Yet, God remains a mystery to me.

Cornelius Plantinga, Jr., in his book *A Sure Thing* says that sometimes we become so familiar with God that we lose the feeling of mystery or awe of Him. He says that sometimes we hear His name so often and worship Him so regularly that, as he puts it, God almost seems like "an unseen uncle who lives in another country." If we are alone at night and hear the wind come mysteriously through the trees, we may think of God. If we attend the funeral of someone we love, we may feel the strangeness of death and the mystery of God. Or suppose we experience cancer and healing, "we may sense an atmosphere that is strange and awesome to us."

A mystery is something puzzling, secret, or unknown to us. We read mystery books, watch mystery movies, and observe mysterious persons. Multiply this a thousand times in thinking of the mystery of God. Even when we love God and trust that God loves us, we still cannot see Him or know everything about Him.

But because of His faithfulness to us, we do know God partly. Through His Word and through His creation, He has let us discover something of who He is and how He wants us to live. We will never understand all of who God is because He is beyond our imagination, but one thing is for sure, we can see that He is good. Good in a sense that is beyond our understanding.

Sometimes we experience unpleasant things. It's during these times that we draw close to God. We think, contemplate, and reflect upon who He is. We experience His closeness and, yes, we feel His mystery.

In Job 11:7 Zophar, the third of Job's friends to chastise him, asks, "Can you fathom the mysteries of God? Can you probe the limits of the Almighty?" Then the book goes on to reveal a mysterious and gracious God, one that Job admits is too big to understand, too mysterious to really know. He ends with, "I know that you can do all things; no plan of yours can be thwarted. You asked, 'Who is this that obscures my counsel without knowledge?' Surely I spoke of things I did not understand, things too wonderful for me to know."

But it isn't only through unpleasant times that we can experience God's mystery. That can happen every day—we just have to look for it. I hope you too are experiencing a wonderful, mysterious God. Look for Him today. In Him.

Monday, December 3, 2007 1:09 a.m.
Welcome to a new week,

- Do not take long showers.
- Do not go for walks.
- Do not put your hands in hot water (aka don't do dishes!)
- Do not open cans or do activities that put pressure on your hands.
- Do not take your pills with Diet Coke.
- Do not take your pills on an empty stomach.

Do not, do not, do not. Why all these "do nots"? Because they make my life more comfortable. They give me, as my oncologist would say, better quality of life. When I follow the "rules," I have less pain, less discomfort. When I don't follow the "rules," heat as well as friction to my palms or soles increases the amount of drug in the capillaries and increases the amount of drug leakage. The leakage of the drug results in redness, tenderness, and possibly peeling of my fingers and soles.

Yesterday, as our minister began reading the Ten Commandments, I turned to Exodus 20 and followed along. I noticed all the "shall nots." Sometimes I see them as a bunch of negative directives. But today, as I compared them to the rules for taking my chemo, I saw how they too improve my life. When I try to live as God has commanded, I have a better quality of life. I have less pain, less discomfort, more peace and contentment.

Tonight I took the last dose of chemo for the week, and now I'll have a week off, but I still have to follow the rules because the chemo stays in my body long after I take it. If I want to limit my pain, I'll follow the "do nots." It's the same with my spiritual life—I have to continue past Sunday to follow God's rules. Deuteronomy 5:32 says: "So be careful to do what the LORD your God has commanded you; do not turn to the right or to the left." You may still experience trials, but God's laws will give you a guide that will direct you, give you peace, and help you live a "quality" life. Have a good day.

Wednesday, December 12, 2007 12:20 a.m.

Hello dear friends,

I've been meaning to write all week, but school has kept me too busy. The period just before finals is always hectic with finishing up class work, completing student registration, checking portfolios, correcting assignments, and attending meetings. I'm thankful that my hands and feet have remained almost pain-free the last few weeks, even after I've started back on chemo. I'm again struggling with fatigue so my life has pretty much consisted of teaching and sleeping. I'm sure that once this rigorous routine comes to an end, I'll have more energy. Of course, this probably won't happen until after I've read 64 philosophy of education statements, 64 foundation of education essay tests, nine assessment projects, 15 Gen 100 essays, and 31 diversity issue essay tests. And to think, some people wonder what I do all day? Anybody looking for part-time work? I'm not complaining because assessment comes with the job, but I must say, I'll be glad when all the grades are in.

Thanks for your constant concern and prayers. More later.

JANUARY - JUNE 2008

Thursday, January 3, 2008 4:34 p.m.

Hello to all my dear friends,

Christmas is over and the new year is already on its way. I'm not sure where the last few weeks have gone, but I do know that all my tests are marked, my grades are in, the gifts are all opened, the tree is down and lying on the lawn waiting to be picked up and hauled away, and I've baked, eaten, and am now thinking about how to take off those extra pounds. I can't believe how much time has lapsed since the last time I visited with you.

First of all, I hope all of you had a wonderful Christmas. I hope that each of you was able to feel God's love during this special holiday. To me it is a beautiful time to reflect on God's astonishing gift, a gift given in love, a gift that goes on giving and giving, a gift that gives us life. I love Christmas so much—it is a special time to remember God's gift and then to share it with others. Sometimes it involves material gifts but more often it is special greetings from folks you don't hear from but once a year, or maybe it's a face-to-face greeting with friends you see only at this time, or it could be the time you take to give warm wishes to those you see often. Whatever the circumstance, it seems that during this time, love seems to worm its way into our hearts and we tend to share it more freely. The day we call Christmas is over, but I hope the things we've experienced over the last few weeks will go on living in all of us and that because of it, we will reflect better the wonderful message that God sent to us.

My year began with a fun celebration with Jerry's family. It's been a long time since many of our nieces and nephews were able to get together so we really enjoyed sharing stories and getting to know their children. I found that bowling with three-to-five-year-olds is really fun!

That was the first day of the new year. The second day involved going to doctors' appointments. I had an 8:00 consultation with the rheumatoidologist who took a lot of blood from me a month ago. She had great news—all the tests showed no major problems with inflammation or degeneration. She suggested I guardedly continue on the anti-inflammatory that she prescribed for me six weeks ago. She suggested taking it only when needed because the medication can cause liver damage and my liver counts were somewhat elevated—nothing to worry about now but extended use could possibly lead to potential problems. That wasn't hard news to take; everyone who knows me, knows how hard it is for me to take medication, so her recommendation is easy for me to live with.

From there I drove to the other side of town where I checked in for a PET scan. I've anxiously looked forward to this procedure for the last two weeks. I've made many plans for the coming semester, things I'm really looking forward to, and I knew that the results of the PET scan were going to tell me if I would be able to go forward with them. When I walked out of the clinic, I had the scan in my hand. Those scans are very easy to read so knowing I had the results, I could pretty much read them, and yet I had to wait for three hours to have someone tell me what they said. This wait was trying, to say the least. At 2:00 Jerry, Josh, and my sister-in-law met me at Dr. Krie's office. I had lab work done, vitals taken, and then waited for what seemed like an eternity for Dr. Krie to come into the exam room. It's odd how a mind works. When Dr. Krie took a while to come in, I was sure she was trying to figure out what treatment I should go on for the next three months. When I heard her footsteps, my heart nearly stopped, but when I saw her face, I knew the news was good. It was unbelievable to hear her say that the scan once again showed no cancer. Not long ago she told me that the statistics were very high for cancer returning, and I should be prepared for dealing with it. Now she suggested that I could wait six months for another PET scan. What joy! What a day to celebrate and thank God for his blessing of remission. What a difference this makes in my life. I can continue to look forward to the dreams I have for work, for my family, for church, and I hope for God's bigger kingdom (more about that later). I, along with my family, give thanks to God for this wonderful news of good health. I'll continue on oral chemo pills as long as I can tolerate them. I'll be on the most aggressive dosage with a little less aggressive time span (one week on, one week off instead of two weeks on and one week off), with strict instructions to not do dishes and to wear sensible shoes. Both of those things seem to agitate the skin on my feet and hands, in that order.

Thanks for all you've given to me the past year. Thanks for keeping me in your prayers, for loving me and my family in so many different ways. God has been good and so have you.

More later. Love to all of you.

Wednesday, March 5, 2008 11:09 p.m.

To my dear friends,

It has been a long time since I've written on this site—two months to be exact. The old adage, how time flies when you are having fun, has surely been true for me the past few months. Life has been full with teaching, observing student teachers, church life, and grandchildren. I'm grateful that I'm able not only to teach this semester but to enjoy every minute of it. God is good. It has taken a bit to figure out my chemo medication but it appears that we are finding the right dosage. I've cut down from 3000 mg to 2000 mg and I've gone to a one-week on, one-week off pattern. With this routine, I don't experience too much pain in my hands and feet. My skin gets a bit dry but lotions and band-aids have helped. I've also learned that I should not plan a lot of activities the weekend after I've taken my medication. I'm usually exhausted and need much sleep. Of course, I'm never sure if it is the chemo or my sleep habits. Once in a while a student will ask me (after they've received a late-night e-mail), if I stay up as late as they do.

As I run into old friends and acquaintances, I'm continually amazed to hear that people continue to pray for me. Thank you! Again, God is good. He continues to lay this on your heart.

Each day I thank God for the restored health He has given me. I'm thankful, grateful, amazed. As I relish this blessing, I'm also aware of the sadness that is evident in the lives of many of my friends. My heart breaks for a friend who has been diagnosed with cancer, another who recently had a recurrence, a friend who lost her job, another who has suffered a significant head injury. When I think of all these hurting people, I hope and pray that they are experiencing God's grace through their trials.

This week my nephew sent a revealing word picture that a coworker shared with him. I found it to be wonderfully comforting. Kathy Bosscher wrote: "So often, living by faith reminds me of floating on water. Unless one stretches out full length and leans back, fully surrendering to the vast undergirding ocean of God's love, we sink." I think of my back floats. I struggle to stay afloat unless I tip my head back and put my ears under the water. I don't necessarily like to feel the water in my ears so I resist until I feel myself sinking. That's when I start to think about what has worked in the past, and I do it. Sometimes I forget how God loves and supports me and I try it on my own. It never works. Kathy continues, "We know full-well that God's love carries the Universe and Grace upholds Time and Eternity, but to lean back? Ah, that is the struggle. And then, there is prayer. Through the prayers of God's people, the Holy

Spirit whispers, 'Lean back. Lean back. Lean on Me.'" What a good reminder for all of us.

You might have noticed the new background. This one is for all my grandsons who love to play soccer (and Amira too). I should also add it's for our son-in-law. He begins his coaching season in a few days. Even in my silence, you've been wonderful. I thank you for your support.

Saturday, March 8, 2008 11:47 p.m.

Dear friends,

On Friday I had an appointment with Dr. Krie. I hadn't seen her for over two months. I've had my blood tested during that period and the tests were always good, so she allowed me to cancel a couple of appointments. At my January appointment she suggested we wait until July for the next PET scan but now she's decided I should have a scan next month so I'm scheduled for one on April 8. I tried to convince Dr. Krie that my feet were doing really well and that I thought I was ready for an increase in dosage so she decided I could maybe increase my pills by one a day. That was before she took a look at my right foot. One look and she said, "No way." I thought my foot was looking pretty good, but she said it was too red and the skin too dry for me to be able to increase the dose. So I'll continue with the same pattern and the dosage that I've been on the past few weeks and continue to pray that this dosage works against the cancer. She also is considering the possibility of having radiation done on my chest wall this summer. It wasn't something I wanted to hear, but I'll definitely do what she thinks is best. A good friend of mine died in January from cancer that moved to her chest wall so if Dr. Krie decides this is a good medical move, I'll do it. One thing we have to consider is that I won't be able to take chemo during this time so Dr. Krie will have to decide if this is a risk we can take.

I continue to thank God for each and every day that I can work and enjoy my family, friends, and students. Each day I think about the psalmist's words in Psalm 118:24: "This is the day that the Lord has made; let us rejoice and be glad in it." As a new week begins, I'm eager to look for the reasons God has given me to live and serve Him. In Him.

Thursday, March 13, 2008 12:17 a.m.

Dear friends,

So many heartaches, so many worries, so many unknowns. Tomorrow our friends are going to welcome a new grandchild into this world. They know he is going to be born with some disabilities; with what they don't know for sure. Tomorrow my nephew will hear the diagnosis of tests that were taken over the weekend. They fear the unknown of the future. Tomorrow my friends who were involved in a car accident will continue to struggle to rebuild their lives. Their family is struggling with the pain of seeing their parents struggle. Tomorrow a friend who is battling cancer hopes to build her white count. So many sad and unknown things. Things that make us worry. It is enough to make one's heart hurt. But then I think of who God is and I'm reminded of how He walked with us over the last year, and I trust that He will walk with them too. God has proven to be faithful; morning by morning we wake up to find His power and His comfort.

Earlier this week I was reminded of His power through a sight I saw as I drove to work. As I turned onto the highway, I was met with a winter whiteness. As I drove down Highway 18, I was surrounded in fog. Not many miles later, I caught the sun rising in my rearview mirror. It was big, and it was orange. What a sight! Shortly after, the sun began to burn off some of the fog. What I saw was the most beautiful picture—the fog lifted from the bottom and from the top, but left a patch of fog in the middle. As I continued down the road, I saw that the middle of the landscape was missing, engulfed in fog. I could see only the bottom third of barns, houses, trees, and the top third. It was an amazing sight! Such a mystery!

It reminded me of the mystery of God's perfect ways. We don't understand His ways but through all the troubles of the world, He shows us who He is—a God who cares for us, in good times and bad. A God who is faithful through all.

The second verse of Sara Groves' song, "He's Always Been Faithful" says what I feel:

> I can't remember a trial or a pain
> He did not recycle to bring me gain
> I can't remember one single regret
> In serving God only, and trusting His hand
> All I have need of, His hand will provide
> He's always been faithful to me.

I pray that all those going through sad times will know and feel God's faithfulness each morning. In Him.

Thursday, March 20, 2008 1:16 a.m.

For those of you who check the time I write, I was in bed but then remembered I had forgotten to take my chemo pills. It is difficult for me to take them, so I put them off until I know I can't avoid them anymore. Tonight I really worked at avoiding them. As long as I was up again, I decided to write on my CaringBridge site.

Earlier tonight I sent out a YouTube video to some friends. It was a video of two teams of Japanese men having a marshmallow eating contest. This was no ordinary contest. The marshmallows were attached somehow above the contestants' heads. The men stood with their backs to a board that had a thick rubber cord attached about nose high. The contestants put the cord around their head, between their mouth and nose and then walked forward, stretching the cord while they tried to reach the marshmallows. I watched the video when I was in my office today. As I watched the contortion of the men's faces as they flexed and pulled so they could grab the treats, I shook with laughter. The sound of my laughter got the only colleague working on my office floor wondering what I was doing. We don't belly laugh often, but we should. Research says it's good for our health.

One research project that I read says that big gulps of oxygen, like the ones we get when we laugh heartily, can destroy cancer cells. Maybe some of you don't worry about that, but the article also said that parasites and bacteria don't survive well in the presence of extra oxygen. Even if you don't believe this, you have to admit that laughter is good for the soul. Some people have taken up the new fad of visiting an oxygen bar (I've seen them in European airports) so they can fill their bodies with more oxygen. It's much cheaper to have a good laugh. The Bible says it's good for us too: "A cheerful heart is good medicine, but a crushed spirit dries up the bones" (Proverbs 17:22).

I hope you find something humorous to laugh about today. In Him.

Sunday, March 23, 2008 1:43 a.m.

Dear friends,

Yesterday I spent a wonderful day with my twin sister and mom. My mom wanted to do some shopping so Marcia and I spent a great day picking out bedding and curtains, selecting new clothes and of course eating. Mom was insistent that we take her to a restaurant that was new to her and that we find a place for a good piece of pie. We had an enjoyable time reminiscing about the past, enjoying the present, and talking about the future. Isn't that what life is about?

As I think about today, Easter Sunday, I think about the past, present, and future too. I remember the past and know that Jesus died for my sins, to pay what I couldn't pay for. Today I live because He lived, died, and rose again. I hope and pray that I am living this life, not in payment for my sins, because I can't do that, but in thanksgiving for this gift of life I have because of grace. And I remember tomorrow, sometime in the future, a time I'll live in glory with Him. What comfort, what peace.

I hope that each of you will not only be able to celebrate today with your loved ones but also take time to remember the greatest gift you've ever been given. Happy Easter.

Monday, March 31, 2008 1:12 a.m.

Hello friends,

I've had quite a weekend. It began already on Thursday. One of our friends bought a taco supper for a group of people from a local restaurant at the benefit auction last spring. They invited us and a bunch of friends to join them. We had a wonderful time celebrating my health and good friendships. I was even given a beautiful bouquet of flowers. It was a lovely night.

On Friday I went with my cousin Kim, my aunt Marilyn, and my mom to the Women of Faith conference in Omaha. It was wonderful. The music was fantastic, the speakers were inspiring, and the company was great. We heard Sandi Patty, Patsy Clairmont, Sheila Walsh, Marilyn Meberg, Max Lucado, and Luci Swindoll. All of them were fabulous, inspiring us through the events that had happened in their lives. One of the messages that came through over and over was the importance of putting our trust in God. Sandi Patty, who was my favorite this weekend, reminded me that sometimes I can't or won't see God but it isn't because God isn't there. He is always there, waiting for me to see Him, but often I'm not looking for Him. Sometimes I get too caught up in solving my own problems, trying to help myself, taking time to figure things out that I forget to go to God. Why? I don't know. He has always shown His faithfulness to me, and yet I often overlook His ability to help me. In II Corinthians 12:9, Paul quotes Jesus as saying, "My grace is sufficient for you, for my power is made perfect in weakness."

I am weak. Sometimes I doubt if I can do my job well enough, I worry that my cancer will pop back up, I question my ability to be an effective mother and grandmother. I fail at all of them at times, but in my failures, I can be assured that God will develop my Christian character and deepen my worship of Him—if I look to Him. When I admit my weakness, I affirm God's strength. I'm thankful that God has sent many people into my life who have helped me in my weaknesses. This weekend was a perfect example of that. Thank you. In Him.

Monday, April 7, 2008 12:16 a.m.

Dear friends,

Sunday was a wonderful day. Our church services were very meaningful. A few Dordt students helped lead our evening worship. They did a fantastic job of helping us feel the majesty and power of God.

As I look toward the week ahead, I feel a bit anxious. My teaching load looks a bit easier. I had a stressful week last week trying to figure out how I could best teach about the philosophy of education. Now that I've done my job, the students will spend this week finding ways to make it relevant to them and their education. Many interesting topics in my other classes come up in Ed. Philosophy so that makes my teaching easier in those classes.

My anxiety this week has nothing to do with school. It has to do with the PET scan that I'm having on Tuesday. It is easy to talk about being confident in God's power to heal, but talk can be cheap. It's not that I don't believe that God can heal, but sometimes it is difficult to believe He will choose to keep the cancer away from me. Every time I've felt a pain in my chest the past couple of weeks, I've worried and considered all the "what ifs."

As I sang the songs with the congregation in church yesterday, I was comforted by many of the words. The second and third verses from "Amazing Grace" were especially meaningful: "The Lord has promised good to me, His Word my hope secures; He will my shield and portion be as long as life endures. Through many dangers, toils, and snares I have already come; 'tis grace hath brought me safe thus far, and grace will lead me home."

Ah, God's grace—it's that free gift that quiets my heart and gives me hope for tomorrow. Praying you have a good week.

Tuesday, April 8, 2008 9:17 p.m.

Hello everyone,

I had an entry ready to go earlier and somehow lost it. We wanted to let you all know that mom had a PET scan again today and again we are rejoicing and praising God because it came back clear! Thank you all for your prayers. Mindy

Wednesday, April 9, 2008 12:20 a.m.

Hello friends,

As you can probably imagine, we are rejoicing with all our beings for the wonderful report that was given to us yesterday. For the past week, both Jerry and I have been very anxious. If we had known what Dr. Krie was worried about, we would have probably been even more anxious. We didn't know that my last blood test showed that my liver count was up, nor did we know that it is very common for someone who has been diagnosed with stage four cancer to have it recur within six months of a clean scan. Dr. Krie explained it this way—I can't explain why the cancer hasn't returned, all I can say is the Man Upstairs is watching out for you. We translated that to say that it is God's will for my life. The end of verse 16 of Psalm 139 says: "All the days ordained for me were written in your book before one of them came to be." Statistics do not know the time-table that God has for my life. I'm glad He is in control and I'm thankful for His healing hand.

Thank you for all your prayers and your words of encouragement. I hope you will join us in thanking God for the remission of the cancer.

In Him. Jerry and Cella

Thursday, April 10, 2008 9:18 p.m.
Dear friends,

I just can't wipe the smile off my face. Somebody asked me today what my scan showed and a friend who was next to me said, "Can't you tell by the smile on her face?"

Barbara Johnson always made me laugh. She had a very serious message that she told with humor. Recently I read something from Barbara Johnson that struck me as true. She said, "Nothing this side of heaven is forever. Hair will be shorn; hair will grow back (usually). Faces will fall, no matter how many times we get them lifted. My losses can't be recouped. The future is unknown. Time changes, we change, everything changes."

Another bottom-line truth comes to mind: "I the Lord do not change" (Malachi 3:6). Whew! Nothing remains the same except God. God's Word is immutable and His Word is final. His stubborn love for us never varies or wavers. Regardless of our losses or the length of our hair, "God's promises are true, and His love holds us fast."

What a blessing to know and believe God's promises!

Continuing to smile and thank God.

Monday, June 2, 2008 1:32 a.m.
Dear friends,

I can't believe it has been so long since I have written on this site. The last weeks of school kept me busy finishing up my classes, grading tests, and preparing for my trip to Nigeria. That is where I am right now. I don't have much time to write, but I wanted you all to know that I'm doing well. I just finished another round of chemo, even while I'm here in Nigeria. I'm feeling really good—even my feet are doing alright. I'm absolutely loving this beautiful warm weather. I'm much happier sweating than freezing. As I said, I don't have much time to write now, but I will try to update with more information in a couple of days. I'm hoping to add some new photos too. In Him.

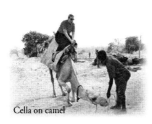

Cella on camel

August - December 2008

Thursday, August 28, 2008 12:05 p.m.

Hello everyone,

I'm sorry we haven't updated for a while. I thought I'd let everyone know that mom found out on Tuesday that she has cancer on her brain. There are two spots—one on the left front and the other on the right side. She will be having surgery tomorrow morning at nine at McKennan to remove the spot on the left front and then we hope will be having radiation. I will let you know how the surgery goes and how she is doing when we know. Thank you for all of your thoughts and prayers. Mindy

Friday, August 29, 2008 3:47 p.m.

Mom's surgery has been finished for a little while and she is doing well. It went very well and took an hour and 30 minutes. The surgeon was happy with how everything went and said that the tumor was 100% removed. Praise the Lord! Mom is in ICU and is resting. She will continue to be in ICU for at least the next 24 hours and if everything looks good with her vitals, should be able to go to a different room tomorrow. Her color looks good and she is very responsive! Thank you for all of your prayers; we definitely have felt them all. Mindy

Saturday, August 30, 2008 2:50 p.m.

Mom is still doing well, but is very tired and needs her rest so we're trying to limit the visitors since she is still in ICU. If you would like to visit with dad or any of the family we would love to see you, but be aware that if you come, you probably won't be able to see her at all. Mindy

Saturday, August 30, 2008 6:02 p.m.

I will write more in a little while, but I wanted to let you know that mom has been moved to the first floor to room 1-152. Mindy

Sunday, August 31, 2008 4:16 a.m.

To my dear friends,

Yes, it is early in the morning and I can't sleep so I thought I would quickly drop a note into the CaringBridge site. Surgery did go well and

I am very thankful for that. We now have to face the future. Early next week we will be making some decisions on the next steps to overcoming this hurdle. We hope the doctors will be able to provide us with great treatment that will bring about full restoration of health. Please continue to pray with us. In Him.

Monday, September 1, 2008 9:14 p.m.

I would like to say thank you to everyone for the prayers they've said and the prayers they continue to say on mom's behalf. Mom's computer is down right now so she'll be on probably tomorrow, but we wanted to let everyone who doesn't know already that she is at home. She was able to go home yesterday already. We could hardly believe that was possible. Again thank you much for all of your prayers. We know this would not be possible without all of you praying and God answering those prayers.

Mindy

Tuesday, September 2, 2008 1:49 p.m.

Dear praying friends,

Thank you to many of you who took the time to pray for me over the past week. I surely wasn't expecting what I just went through. I've been struggling with headaches and loss of words for over a month but after the clear PET scan we decided it was just chemo brain. I'm thankful that the doctors could find the cause of this discomfort so quickly and relieve what I was going through. I'm feeling much better already. Not having those intense headaches and not having to struggle for words is a relief. I'll try to post more later but just wanted all of you to know that I am very grateful for competent and caring doctors and wonderful, praying friends. In Him.

Saturday, September 6, 2008 9:26 p.m.

Dear friends,

First of all, thanks to all of you for your support for us over the past week and a half. It is hard for me to be able to put into words how I am feeling. The first bout of cancer was hard but this has been much more difficult. I know I was always told the cancer would likely return but I wasn't quite ready for this news, especially after the clear PET scan. I'm thankful for the successful surgery. What a blessing to have surgeons who are competent! I couldn't imagine how wonderful I felt after surgery. So of course, I did too much. My brain swelled some which was a good reminder for me to take it easy. I've worked very hard the past few days to sit as quiet as I could. I had people come and help with things so I had no excuse to be moving around. Now I'm looking forward to seeing the radiologist-oncologist on Monday. I hope she will be able to design the head gear that will be used for whole-head radiation. At that time she will also consult with us as to when treatment will begin. We are hoping it will be very soon. I'll keep you posted.

I am thankful to God for all He has provided—doctors, nurses, friends, family. I hope you will continue to pray with us that God will bring healing. Thank you.

Sunday, September 7, 2008 10:46 p.m.

Dear friends,

To be honest with you, I've been feeling a little down the past few days. The first cancer diagnosis was difficult, but this second one has been much more difficult. I find myself feeling sorry for myself and asking why me. And then I realize, why not me. The journal entries you entered the past few days have helped to pick me up and bring my hope back. I thank you very much for the encouragement, the prayers, the love you have shown.

Tomorrow morning we leave to have my head-gear designed and then we will, I hope, get my schedule for the radiation treatments. I am hoping to begin very soon. Jerry isn't as hopeful as I am that we could begin already this week. Please pray along with us that I will be able to accept what the doctor recommends. Again, thanks so much for your support, love, and care. We couldn't go through this alone. Thanks for the reminders that God is in control and that He never leaves us nor forsakes us. We feel His comfort at this time. In Him.

Monday, September 8, 2008 3:56 p.m.

Hello dear praying friends,

Just a quick update to let you know that we had a wonderful check-up with the radiologist-oncologist today. I had my head-gear designed and then heard the great news that I can begin radiation tomorrow. In case this would happen, I had grabbed a few clothes before we left so that I can stay up here a few days and avoid the travel from Sanborn to Sioux Falls.

Thanks for all your prayers! I'll write more a little later.

Monday, September 8, 2008 8:25 p.m.

Dear friends,

I've been trying hard to process all that has happened to me the past couple of weeks. I'm still working at it, but the e-mail I received from Megan has helped me a lot. I thought you might enjoy it too:

I will never forget a question I had with someone when I was at Dordt, I think my sophomore year. I was starting to process all that happened to Josh and our family as a result. And I asked this person why it had to happen to our family. And he responded "why not?" At first, I was stunned—and then angry. I couldn't believe he dared ask that question because . . . well, because . . . well . . . I never did come up with an answer. It really truly got me thinking. Why not our family? Because we believed? Because we were good people? Because we went to church every Sunday? Because we did service projects? It made me realize that all the good things in life we experience are God's grace, freely given to us. We don't deserve protection or shielding of pain because we are Christians. Sin is everywhere, permeating even our inner core. And yet, God gives us goodness. He gives us joy, good news, and does indeed protect us. Sometimes we can twist that around to mean that nothing bad will happen to us, but we miss the point if that is our focus. When we focus on the grace still extended, even amidst the storms, we can still live a life of thanks. We don't deserve to be protected and yet God protects. And in His infinite wisdom, he knows how to protect us when we think we are just flailing in the storm.

When you were first diagnosed, I did ask the question of why, not in doubt that God wasn't taking care of us, but wondering what He could be cooking up. It got me reflecting to years back when you were diagnosed with cervical cancer, before I had any memory. It dawned on me that God could have taken you home to Him then, but He knew you were needed to raise and form your children and the community. And it made me very thankful. I wouldn't be who I am without your influence. And it made me wonder how many other times I hadn't noticed God doing the very best thing for us as we passed through one day at a time, sometimes not acknowledging His ever-present care.

Sometimes we get answers to the whys we have in life and other times we do not. I wondered why about the timing of this baby, and now having to go home and not having to decide if we do or not—it answered some of my questions. We may not know the why of your two diagnoses with cancer, mom. But I do know that you have formed our community and our family. God has used you in powerful ways. And He will continue to, if you are in the classroom or resting on the couch. Countless people love you and countless listen to the words you have to say as you bravely and honestly and faithfully walk this journey of cancer. People can see your strong faith when they first meet you. It's okay to have down days and it's okay to be scared and sad. But knowing you, even those moments will be flavored with faith, a steady reliance on the God you love and serve.

When I think about why, I admit that I used to think "good" people deserved "good" things. This journey you are walking really wasn't intended by God for anyone to travel, but how much better for a Christian with a living hope to travel this journey than someone who lives for the moment.

Thanks for letting me share.

Tuesday, September 9, 2008 11:25 a.m.
Dear friends,

A quick update to let you know I survived my first radiation treatment. It was painless and effortless. They attached the head-gear to my head and then zapped me on each side of the head with the radiation. It does feel a little weird to have a plastic mask tight over your face, but I'm not complaining. Thanks for your prayers.

Wednesday, September 10, 2008 3:01 p.m.
Dear friends,

Two treatments down and thirteen to go! My second treatment went very well. The technicians are very informative and encouraging. I met with the PA and the radiologist-oncologist today and was very encouraged by their reports. Basically, I will receive the 15 treatments and then wait approximately one month for an MRI to determine what the treatments did to the tumor that is remaining. So for right now, I fervently ask that you pray that the tumor will shrink, but even more that it will disappear. God asks us to ask boldly and that is what I intend to do. I humbly ask you to do this with me.

We feel blessed to be surrounded by such a cloud of witnesses, faithful prayer warriors who hold us up before our Father in heaven. Thank you for your wonderful support.

Thursday, September 11, 2008 9:22 a.m.
Good Morning,

I'm writing a little earlier in the day, but it's looking like a busy day so I thought I'd update you. Today is the day I see the neurologist. He will more than likely take out my stitches, go over reports, give some advice and prognosis. I'm eager to hear what he has to say. One question I have is about the tumor that still remains in my head. How is it affecting me now? Or is it? Sometimes I wonder if the things I think I am noticing are real or different from before. I appreciated him during our visits in the hospital, so I'm looking forward to his visit today. After that I will be going for a 3:00 p.m. radiation treatment. As of now, the rest of my treatments are set up for this time. Jerry will then take me home and I'll drive up for my Friday treatment with a friend.

We are thankful for how things have worked out. Again, like last time, we had minimal waiting for any test or procedure. What a blessing! It may not make much difference as far as physical health, but it surely helps with my mental health.

I know that we as a family are feeling much more encouraged than when we began this whole thing. It comes down to the grace of God and how He manifested it through His wonderful caring people. Thanks much for whatever part you have played in this journey. In Him.

Friday, September 12, 2008 12:25 p.m.

Dear friends,

In a little while I'll be leaving for my fourth treatment. Today I'll be traveling from Sanborn. It will be a longer trip but it was very good to get home. I had a wonderful stay by my sister-in-law and brother-in-law (in fact, I felt quite pampered). They were gracious in providing me with great care.

My appointment yesterday went well. The doctor told me that the tumor that remains is fairly deep. Of course, I right away worried that the radiation wouldn't hit it, but he assured me that radiation goes through inches of lead so it would surely hit the tumor. He was so pleased with what he saw that he dismissed me for now. That felt good! He did tell me that it will more than likely take a while for the tumor in my head to shrink or die so I will probably continue to notice some side effects like my left eye fluttering and the occasional blurring of my right eye. I may also notice a little weakness on my right side. I'll have another MRI about one month after the radiation is completed. If the tumor is slow-growing the cells reproduce slower, so if we do the MRI too soon, we won't see the results. So much to learn.

The radiation treatment was fast. They didn't have to do x-rays this time so it was a matter of zapping me.

I often wonder how I could take this journey by myself. You have all been tremendously encouraging! You have lifted me up in ways I couldn't imagine. To tell you the truth, this did hit me hard. I thought I was pretty well on my way to beating this thing, so it was a blow to hear the news of a brain tumor. This site, the cards, the personal contacts have all helped me to see this as a way to look to God for my strength. It is again a way for me to see the power of God—through His beautiful people!

I want to say thanks—thanks from the bottom of my heart. I'm very glad to be a part of the family of God. In Him.

Saturday, September 13, 2008 7:18 a.m.

Good Morning friends,

Last night I was surfing through the net, my e-mails, Dordt's home page, etc. I read some things about brain tumors and decided that was too scary to continue, so I moved on to the special features on Dordt's home page. I clicked on a few things and then turned to the article about James Schaap's new book. I hope you don't mind me mentioning this, Jim. Jim has just finished a devotional book on the Psalms called *Sixty at Sixty: a Boomer Reflects on the Psalms*. I've mentioned before that this new development with cancer has been difficult to accept but something in the article reminded me once again of the powerful God I serve. Here it is: "As noted in a devotional based on Psalm 37:18, 'the picture of open, warm and loving hands extended to us each morning is the assurance, simply stated, that God knows. God's not off on a cruise or so wrapped up with the crisis in Iraq that he has no time for our problems.'" I do not know what the future holds as far as my disease, but I do know that He holds it. I know that He cares for me and will never leave or forsake me or my family. For that I am grateful!

Can you believe it? I'm one-third of the way through my treatments. From Sanborn it seems a long way to go for a couple minutes of zapping, but I'm definitely not complaining. I am grateful for modern technology. As I lie there, strapped to the table, I marvel at the machine that radiates the killing rays to the tumor in my head and yet passes by the good cells. I'd surely like to thank those who developed this treatment. I'm thankful for all those who have agreed to give me rides. I'm very appreciative of their willingness to give of their time. I have two days off now and will begin again on Monday.

Again, thanks much for all the ways you encourage us. Thanks for your prayers, your notes, the flowers, the gifts of money, everything! You are the best.

Sunday, September 14, 2008 9:39 p.m.

Dear praying friends,

It was a great weekend. Jerry has been trying to keep me as quiet as possible, but over the past few days he's loosened the reins a little. On Saturday we had the privilege of going to a very good friend, Seth O.'s, wedding. It was a late afternoon outdoor wedding. The scenery was beautiful as was the ceremony. We had a good time visiting with friends, especially the Oostenink family. It felt good to be part of life once again. I'm eager to move on. Yes, I know, I have a bit to go before I can put this behind me, but bit by bit I'm going to make it. Next week I'll be getting treatments every day. I'm also planning on going back to Dordt to begin getting back to work. I'm eager to meet my students whom I've not yet met and begin sharing with them the excitement of the teaching profession. That is a prayer concern—that I have enough energy to accomplish the plans I have made. The only side effect I really need to be concerned with is a bit of fatigue as treatments continue. And there is one other, since I'm receiving whole-head radiation, I'll once again lose my hair. I'm not concerned about the hair—it's kind of nice not to have to do my hair each day—I think it's more the loss, a loss I have no control over. But if I can get healthy again, the hair is really nothing. The doctor tells me that my hair will come in even slower than after chemo treatments so it might be December before I see hair on my head again. Oh well, hats, here I come!

God is good! I know many of you have mentioned this on my site, as have I in the past. But I really mean it. Once again I'm thrown into a time where I really have to rely on God. Many of you know our life history and how it seems that if it can happen, it will happen to the Bosmas. Sometimes I ask God if He doesn't think I've had enough to make me rely on Him, enough to put my trust in Him. I don't know His for-sure-answer, but through all of these circumstances I've come to realize that God doesn't wish these things for us. God isn't the one who creates the pain and suffering. But He is the one who comforts. He is the one who brings peace. He is the one who cares, cares enough to instill in others a desire to help and care for us. All I can say is "Thank you, God. Thank you for your abiding love."

Have a good week.

Tuesday, September 16, 2008 12:14 a.m.

For the past week I've been walking. I love walking in the country and since we live just one house from a gravel road, it is very easy to slip out there for a mile walk. (Yeah, I know Pat and Cath, it isn't a marathon but it is exercise.) As I walk I have time to reflect on life, sometimes with more positive thoughts than others. Today as I walked my beaten path, I was really struck by the changing of the seasons. Since I love the heat, the fall season isn't necessarily my favorite because it is the season that reminds me that winter is coming. But it is also the season that gives me a good picture of God, the creator of all things. On Sunday I heard a sermon based on Genesis 1. When I saw the text, I wondered if I was going to hear an interpretation of how the world was created but I was pleasantly surprised to hear Pastor Greg talk about God creating the world to show us who He is and to give us an opportunity to glorify Him. Now as I walked I noticed the beans change from their beautiful, fresh green color to their rich, golden hues and I am reminded of God. A God who is in perfect control of what is happening in nature. A God who knows just what has to happen for a bean plant to be harvested. He takes care of every little detail. What a reminder that if God takes care of every little creational detail, He surely is taking care of every little person too. What a comfort to know that God knows about me and you, that He holds us in His hand and carries us through every trial that comes our way.

"This is what God the LORD says—he who created the heavens and stretched them out, who spread out the earth and all that comes out of it . . . . I the Lord, have called you in righteousness; I will take hold of your hand. I will keep you and will make you to be a covenant for the people and a light for the Gentiles . . . " (Isaiah 42:5, 6).

Today's treatment lasted the typical couple of minutes. The technicians are pleasant and informative which makes the treatments easier. Tomorrow's appointment will include a doctor's consultation and probably x-rays so it will be a bit longer. I also am going back to Dordt tomorrow. I plan to observe a class that I will begin teaching on Thursday. I'm really excited but nervous. Can I do it? Can I learn the students' names? Will my memory allow me to remember the things I need to remember? Please pray for a good memory and enough stamina to teach and continue the trips to Sioux Falls.

Have a good day.

Tuesday, September 16, 2008 10:31 p.m.

Dear uplifting friends,

After I returned home from my treatment today, I grabbed the mail off the table and sat down to read it. I was once again amazed, humbled, in awe, overjoyed, astonished, excited (what else can I add) as I read through the beautiful cards that I received. I can't believe that so many of you continue to remember and pray for me. What a blessing you have all been! I can't begin to thank you for all you have done and continue to do for us. You remind me of the tribes that Joshua was talking to after they settled in Canaan. In chapter 22:5 he compliments them for their obedience and then gives them the command to "love the LORD your God, to walk in his ways, to obey his commands, to hold fast to him and to serve him with all your heart and all your soul." That's what I see in you.

Today's treatment was once again quick. I went into the room (a room with six-foot walls of concrete, lay down, put on my face mask, got my mask bolted to the table, got zapped on each side of my head, and then I was finished. Today I saw the PA and the radiologist-oncologist. They administered a neurological test which they said I passed with flying colors. I'm continuing to pray that God is allowing the radiation I'm receiving to kill the tumor and any other cells that might still remain. I hope you will continue to pray with me. Thanks.

Wednesday, September 17, 2008 9:41 p.m.

Dear faithful prayer warriors,

My treatment today went as usual. Quick and easy. I did have an x-ray to make sure the radiation is hitting the right areas but that took only a few seconds. I'm still not too excited about these trips to Sioux Falls. But I've surely met many fantastic people while in treatment—kind, caring, informative. God has put amazing people in my life, including all of you.

I haven't been sleeping well since surgery so today we stopped and picked up some Tylenol PM. I'm hoping that will help. Today I cut down on the Decadron I've been taking. My brain may swell some with the treatments, so the doctor wants me to continue with the drug for awhile but at a lesser dose. I'm halfway with my treatments. Well, almost; I've just completed my seventh treatment and have eight to go. Isn't that fantastic?

Tomorrow I will begin teaching my very first class of the semester. I am excited! I can't wait to get to know the students and help introduce them to the wonderful world of teaching. I'm very thankful for my colleagues who have so ably taken my classes thus far. They have been a blessing in my life. God does provide in amazing ways. Thank you to all of you who have and to some who are still helping me!

Thanks for your support.

Thursday, September 18, 2008 8:56 p.m.

Dear friends,

Oh, what a beautiful mornin',
Oh, what a beautiful day.
I got a beautiful feelin'
Ev'rything's goin' my way.

As I rode down the highway today, the lyrics of this old song ran through my mind. It was a wonderful day! Wonderful because the weather was beautiful. Wonderful because I was in the company of good friends. Wonderful because it was my first day back teaching. Is there anything better? It was great to be back in class. My students were wonderful. Even though I taught freshmen and they don't really know me, they were eager to have me in class. What a way to energize a person. I'm thankful for work and for my students.

But now I'm tired; it was a long day. The treatment again went very well, in and out as usual. Again today we received food and encouraging cards. Thank you much for all the things you do to encourage us. In Him.

Saturday, September 20, 2008 12:57 a.m.

Dear friends,

Maybe "everything going my way" wasn't exactly accurate. Those were the last line of the words of the song I quoted yesterday. Today wasn't exactly as I expected. I didn't have class today so I spent the morning working on some lectures and planning for next week. By the time I left for my treatment I could feel pressure in my head; it felt as if I had a tight cap on my head and my eyes were once again fuzzy. I hadn't felt that for quite a while. My treatment went well, but the radiology technicians decided I should see the doctor to try to figure out how I could get rid of the extra pressure. The doctor decided I should probably go back to taking three doses of Decadron once again. That means I'll probably be taking some sleeping pills to help me sleep. I can live with that. One of the side effects of radiation is brain swelling, so it isn't atypical that I am experiencing this. I continue to learn lessons, one being I'm not in control of what happens to me. Yes, I can seek medical advice; I can choose to follow that advice, but once again I'm seeing that my dependence is on God. Each thing I face reminds me to "Trust in the Lord with all (my) heart and lean not on (my) own understanding; in all (my) ways acknowledge him and he will make (my) paths straight" (Proverbs 3:5).

I do feel much better after taking the additional dose of Decadron so I hope that will take care of the problem.

Thanks once again for your prayers.

Sunday, September 21, 2008 8:08 p.m.

Dear friends,

It was a good weekend. On Saturday I relaxed and did some planning for next week. On Sunday I actually played for the morning service. I was a little afraid of it not going well, but it went just fine. My friend Catherine played viola with me so that made it much easier. We had a wonderful dinner with my family and then I crashed. I can tell that the extra dose of Decadron has really helped the swelling in my head. I no longer experience the blurring of my eyes. Although that has improved, my feet have decided to act up. Over the past 24 hours, they've started to peel. I'm able to pull big hunks of thick skin off my right foot. I'm not sure what this is all about. Maybe it is the result of the Xeloda I was on previously. I'll have to ask the doctor about that this week.

Today I started reading a book that was recommended to me by quite a few people. It's titled *The Shack*. I'm only halfway through it but I'm finding it intriguing. It isn't your typical look at the Trinity, but it definitely is giving me a fresh look at it. *The Shack* is a story about a guy whose young daughter was abducted and murdered while they were camping. He gets a note in his mailbox inviting him to come back to the shack where she was murdered and there he meets the Trinity. Although I haven't finished the book, I'm definitely seeing a God who cares for His children; a God who loves us and wants us to live our life in Him. Sometimes I fall into "Why do I have to go through this? Why me?" And then I read, "I'm not merely the best version of you that you can think of. I am far more than that, above and beyond all that you can ask or think."

Syd Hielema in his review of the book in *The Banner*, our church's publication, says, "The repeated insistence on the fundamental paradox that we are called to know a God who is ultimately unknowable is humbly liberating." Although the book is fiction, it does give us much to think about. It teaches us about a God, as Job said, who is really too big for us to understand, but one we can trust and put our confidence in. I'm trusting in Him as I wait for the radiation to work on the remaining tumor. Please continue to pray with us. Thank you.

Monday, September 22, 2008 9:36 p.m.

Dear friends,

Can you believe it? Ten days down and only five more to go! The time has gone fast but I'm eager for the trips to be finished. Class went well today, at least from my perspective and I had a great driver, my neighbor Phyllis. We had good conversation and the weather was beautiful. One of my students has been hospitalized due to a mass that they found in her abdomen so we had the opportunity to stop a minute and wish her well as she waits for tests tomorrow. She looked and sounded anxious, and I wanted to assure her that God has her in His hands and He will carry her through this trial.

My feet, especially my right foot, look better tonight. My vision is quite clear and I still have hair. I keep tugging at small pieces, checking to see if it is beginning to fall out. But it is rooted well.

Tonight I worked on some lectures for the coming week. It feels good to feel productive. (Maybe I'm not, but it's all in the perception, right?) I'm thankful that I am able to continue to work. Teaching is truly a wonderful profession, one that brings much joy. I hope all of you also feel joy in your work. Years ago we had a minister who often stated that if you did not find joy in your work, you had two options—one was to change your attitude and the other was to change your job. I believe he was right! God calls us to work joyfully for Him in His kingdom. He expects us to love what we do and glorify Him through our work. That's difficult to do when you're dissatisfied with what you are doing. I praise God every day for my job, for my colleagues, for my students, for Dordt College. I hope you too are finding as much joy in your work as I am in mine. Thanks for all your love and care.

Tuesday, September 23, 2008 8:58 p.m.

To my praying friends,

Eleven down and four to go! But who's counting. Again today the treatment went well, in and out in just a few minutes. The trip goes fast when you have a great friend to converse with. Thanks Pat! I'm really looking forward to the end of the treatments, but then the waiting will begin. It will be four to six weeks before they will schedule an MRI so I'll have to wait patiently until we know the results of the treatments. It was explained this way to me—fast-growing tumors reproduce fast, and slow-growing tumors reproduce slowly. Makes sense doesn't it? So if I have an MRI too soon, we could not see accurate results of the treatments. So patience. Not always easy but definitely possible with God by my side. I believe He is all-powerful enough to heal me so I will wait patiently for the radiation to do its work. Some of you have probably had to or are experiencing dealing with impatience too. It isn't always easy, but scripture, friends and family, good books, devotionals, and prayer make it all bearable. In Colossians 1:11, Paul reminds us that we are " . . . being strengthened with all power, according to his glorious might, so that you may have great endurance and patience, and joyfully giving thanks to the Father, who has qualified you to share in the inheritance of the saints in the kingdom of light." What a blessing to be a part of that inheritance. I hope you too are feeling that inheritance and thanking God for it. In Him.

Wednesday, September 24, 2008 10:19 p.m.

Good Evening,

Well, it finally happened. Last night my hair began to fall out. I could pull it out by little tufts. Tonight I had Mindy buzz what remained, so it is back to hats and scarves. I'm trying to tell myself the positives and thinking about the cup being half full (instead of being half empty). For one, it doesn't take long to get ready in the morning when you don't have to do your hair. Some of you have asked about my feet. My right foot isn't looking too good right now but we are thinking that it is the Xeloda working its way out of my system. They don't really hurt but they look pretty awful—red and scaly. I keep applying lotion and covering them with socks.

I've been asked to pray in chapel at Dordt tomorrow. As I was thinking about what to say and doing some reading, I ran across the story of the leper and it was such a good reminder for me in the situation I'm finding myself. The book I was reading is titled *Why Pray?* by John F. De Vries. The title of the chapter was "Dare." The story is found in the book of Matthew and it follows the Sermon on the Mount. The leper, who was an outcast, broke through the crowd to come to Jesus. Can you imagine how angry some of those healthy people must have felt? He was supposed to stay on the outside of society, not be there among the healthy people. Jesus had done some miracles but He had never healed a leper. What made the leper think that he could be healed of this stinking, rotting disease? But he had faith. He barged into the crowd and approached Jesus. But there is something amazing about this—even though he was daring, he was also humble. He says, "If you are willing, you can make me clean." He comes with great faith. Saying this, he indicates that he knows Jesus can heal him if He wants to even though He hasn't done this before.

He then kneels and worships Christ. Humble and daring! A faith-filled daring! He risks everything because he feels passionately about Christ's ability to heal him.

What a story! What an encouragement to me. I too come daring, and I pray humbly before God to ask Him to take the cancer out of my brain and my body. I believe, like the leper, that this is not too much to ask of God. I come boldly knowing He can heal me. I come humbly, knowing it is His will that will be done.

Once again, thanks for all the ways you encourage me. Today I had lunch with my grandson Bailey at Hull Christian, and I was encouraged by all my friends at the school. Thanks! In Him.

Thursday, September 25, 2008 11:34 p.m.

Good evening dear friends,

One more down and that leaves only two to go. I can't believe I'm this far. It has truly gone faster than I ever expected. Today a good friend, a friend that has been with me through thick and thin, took me for my treatment. It was good to talk about old times and the fun we've had in the past. I loved catching up on her family, especially her grandchildren. We haven't taken much time over the past few years to stay in touch. That happens sometimes, doesn't it. It isn't that we mean to drift apart, but because of circumstances and other activities it happens, but friendship doesn't waver and it doesn't lose track of someone you care about. Proverbs 17:17 says, "A friend loves at all times." The NIV says that a true friend is someone who is available to help in times of distress or personal struggles. I've really felt the friendship of true friends through this all. Thank you to all of you who have reached out in many different ways. Another lesson learned through this experience.

Thanks for how wonderfully you've displayed your friendship to me.

Saturday, September 27, 2008 7:54 a.m.

Dear friends,

Wow, what a day! I guess I never expected it to be such a big day. After teaching a class, I finished up some things in my office and then left with my cousin Kim and my twin sister Marcia for lunch. We had a great time eating and chatting. We stopped at a few stores and then I had my treatment. It went well. Yes, only one more treatment left! After the treatment we left for home and I expected to arrive at home, go to dinner with our good friends Nate, Catherine, and Chyann, and then watch a movie with them. When we arrived at home, I took off my head scarf (telling Jerry that my head was sore and it needed some air), and started for the door. Jerry was insistent that I try my hat on again so he could see how it looked, but I told him my head was too sore. Well, I got almost to the door and I heard a great big "Surprise!" Needless to say, I quickly slipped my scarf on my head and peeked in to see what was going on. I was shocked to see a house full of friends ready to help me celebrate my birthday. It was a great night of celebration and repeating over and over how wonderful it was to celebrate my birthday. What a night! Thanks to all of you who took the time to come and celebrate my birthday with me! Thanks to all of you who wished me birthday greetings through personal greetings, cards, e-mails, face book entries, and in thought.

My head is feeling somewhat burned, especially close to the hair line. But with one treatment to go, I'm okay with it. I am eager to be finished with the trips, even though I did have great drivers with whom I had great conversations. I'm thankful for all the people who were willing to take their time to drive me. Please continue to pray with me that the treatments will now do what they are designed to do, and that I will have patience as I wait for the next MRI.

Thanks for all your encouragement.

Monday, September 29, 2008 6:50 a.m.

Good Morning friends,

Today is my last treatment. I can't believe it. It really went much faster than I anticipated. All those great drivers and being able to teach really helped the time go fast. Over the weekend I was quite fatigued, my head itched and felt very tight due to swelling, and my right foot peeled but I woke up this morning feeling much better. I had hoped to write more last night but I was too fatigued. This morning I have to get some work done so this entry will be short. I'll post more soon.

I do very much appreciate all of you.

Tuesday, September 30, 2008 6:45 a.m.

Dear praying friends,

Yahoo! My treatments are finished! Now the wait begins. The doctor told me today that the radiation can continue to work for at least two more weeks and possibly longer. On Friday I will see Dr. Krie, my oncologist, and we will talk about scheduling the next MRI and what the next step will be in my treatment plan. The last time we talked, she mentioned she had heard of a new drug that I could possibly go on so I'm eager to hear more about it. I know that I will have to be given a special measure of patience until I can have the MRI. The scan won't be for at least six weeks and possibly eight weeks. But I've gotten this far and I realize that I have to give the radiation time to work now. At first I thought there would be a possibility that the tumor would be gone, but the doctor explained to me that there will always be some kind of shadow in the area of the tumor that remains. That was good to know. At least that won't be a surprise to me when we get the results.

Our minister is giving a series of sermons based on the beginning chapters of Genesis. When he began the sermons, I was a little worried we were going to hear some science lessons, but I've been pleasantly surprised at the direction the sermons have taken. For example, this week Pastor Greg preached on the third chapter. Instead of debating who was to blame for sin entering the world, he focused on what our responsibility is now that there is sin. One thing really struck me—he suggested that this passage should be a reminder for us to speak honestly. How often doesn't someone ask us how we are doing and we answer, "Just fine?" That's easy for me to do too. And until recently I did feel pretty fine, but now as I finish my treatments, if I'm honest, I must say I'm very tired. As I walk up the steps to my office, I hope I can make it up with my heavy bags. My legs feel like weights as I take each step upward, my head itches and my throat is dry, my mouth has a large sore in it, my right foot continues to peel, and I still deal with swelling of the brain. I may experience this for another week or two and then I hope the side effects of the radiation and the medication will subside. I'm not complaining, but many of you have asked me how you can pray and these are some specifics for which I would love for you to lift me up to God. I know the side effects won't go away like a zap, but just dealing with them and finding ways to work through them would be helpful.

Did I say, "Thank You" to all of you who made my birthday so special last weekend? It was a wonderful day. If I haven't gotten around to thanking you personally, please accept this as my thank you. The gifts, cards, personal conversations, meant much to me.

Hoping you will continue to pray.

Friday, October 3, 2008 8:01 a.m.

Good Morning friends,

I almost missed a fantastic day! Yesterday was the first day of the Heartland Teachers' Convention. I had decided not to go because I have load of correcting to do, and I knew that it would feel good to stay at home and catch up on rest. Well, after my decision to stay at home,

Anne called and asked if I would be one of the special speakers' contact persons and I couldn't say no. Really, I am getting better at saying no to things, but I couldn't pass this up. It was a great decision. First of all the key speaker was one of the best I have ever heard. David Smith is intelligent, well-schooled, funny, personable; he seems to have it all. His presentation was titled "The Garden of Delight." He began by telling us that his speech was going to be gloriously impractical but it wasn't. It had all kinds of application for teachers and for anyone who is a Christian. I had never thought of living in a garden of delight. I thought the garden of delight was a thing of the past, a thing that disappeared when Adam and Eve left the garden. But that is not so. Yes, we live in an imperfect world. We live with sin all around us. But we also live in the garden and God still continues to water that garden and take care of it. David Smith referred to Genesis 2:15, Ecclesiastes 2:4-9, Psalm 104:16, Psalm 1:3 and Isaiah 5. I hope you can take the time to look them up. He reminded us that the purpose of life is pleasure for God, creation, and ourselves. We need to rejoice when we bring about pleasure through or to these things, but in order to do that we have to have right relationships to God, creation, others and ourselves. What a mandate—to enjoy God's world—have pleasure in it—work toward shalom. I hope all of you experience pleasure in the right sense as you live each day.

After the conference today, I'll be seeing Dr. Krie. I'm eager to have some direction in the new path I will now follow. I'm also eager to ask her some questions such as why do my ears hurt so much? Will my right foot get better soon?

I'll let you know how I turn out. Thanks again for your love and care.

Saturday, October 4, 2008 9:25 a.m.

Hi all,

I meant to send this out yesterday, but the day was so busy, I didn't get an opportunity. It was another wonderful day. Hearing David Smith speak on what it means to be a Garden of Delight in the classroom was exciting. I can't imagine that everyone didn't walk away excited and eager to go back to the classroom. I then had a lovely lunch with my mom before I went to see Dr. Krie.

My appointment went well. We didn't do much planning, mostly because we don't know what is happening. The MRI was set for Nov. 17 so now it is the waiting game. Please pray with us as we wait patiently for that time to come. She is puzzled that my right foot is still peeling and red but thinks it must be the aftereffects of Xeloda. The inside of my ears still burn, but the Aloe Vera cream seems to soothe them. My forehead is peeling but the pain is less, so I think that is beginning to heal too.

As I said in my last entry, I really wasn't planning to go to the conference; I wasn't sure I was ready to see and talk to the many people I would know at the conference. What a mistake it would have been to miss it—not only because of the inspiration, but because of the opportunity to meet and talk with friends. I sometimes forget that I'm making it through all of this because of all of you! I was able to talk to many former students. What a blessing to be able to talk with you! I was able to connect with many good teacher friends from the past. The hugs and words of encouragement were unbelievably uplifting. I'm glad I didn't miss this opportunity.

Proverbs 17:17 says, "A friend loves at all times, . . . " I felt true friendship this weekend. As we struggle through this battle with cancer, we are encouraged by many of you, whether it be through personal words, notes, or other acts of kindness. Thank you. In Him.

Sunday, October 5, 2008 9:58 p.m.
Dear friends,

To be honest with you, even though I thoroughly enjoyed my weekend activities, I fell into a little pity party this weekend. As I talked with friends and relatives, I noticed they all had hair (at least the women); no one else complained of the inside of their ears burning; and I didn't see anyone with a peeling forehead. Again I found myself asking, "Why me?" I know we've talked about why not me, but sometimes it is hard when I look around and see everyone going along as they please and wishing I could do the same. This weekend Janie dropped over a book called *It's All Grace—the best of Eppinga,* a book that is a collection on Richard Eppinga's columns that he wrote in *The Banner* for 40 years. The column was called, "Of Cabbages and Kings." The writings give tidbits of information that encourage readers in their spiritual lives. The entries were easy to read and soon I was up to #6. It was titled "Why Me?" Ha! That caught my attention. In the short passage he turned the "Why me?" to say that even though I suffer from kidney stones, I've been blessed to be raised in a Christian home, been able to eat three square meals a day, and been blessed with much more. Why me? Only because of God's grace. Rev. Eppinga went on to tell the story of Arthur Ashe, a skinny kid from Virginia, who grew up to be the #1 tennis player in the world. In 1988 he received the news that he had contracted AIDS through a blood transfusion. He died in 1993 and asked, "Why me?" Not complaining about his illness but instead thanking God for all His blessings. Why me? Why was I given the opportunity to be raised by Christian parents, to have the joy of a wonderful brother and sister, to be able to have great friends, to enjoy success in school and in other activities, and on and on. Only by God's grace. So often we forget about our blessings. I'm thankful for that short story that reminded me to ask with joy, "Why me?"

I hope you can all ask "Why me?" and be able to thank God for all your blessings. In Him.

Tuesday, October 7, 2008 9:32 p.m.

My dear friends,

I just received the most astonishing e-mail. It came via Megan and I'd like to share it with you.

Dear Mike and Megan,

A year and a half ago, my daughter Carin started a non-profit quilting organization in memory of her grandma, my mom, Margaret Herrema. Our goal is to give quilts to people or organizations who we feel could use some hope and comfort in their lives. After my mom's murder, our family found hope in the promises of scripture, friendships, churches, family, new grandchildren. We were comforted by many and we did not lose hope.

Now we would like to send two quilts that are made out of the same fabric and in the same pattern to you and Megan's mom. Obviously, they can't replace a hug or kiss on the cheek as you visit each other in person, but maybe knowing that you have one and Cella has one that looks and feels the same may be comforting as you continue to be far apart.

When Carin started this program, we asked people to send us their extra fabric. And they did— you should see my basement! Then we asked people to sew for us periodically, and they did. Then Carin and I got busy finishing the quilt tops and sending them out. So far we have given away 31 quilts since August 2007.

I've brought your quilt to Patti at the CRWM office and she gave me your mom's address. I hope your quilt will be on its way soon, and I plan to send the other one to Iowa on Wed. Or Thurs. Our prayers continue for all of you.

I don't even know these people and here they are, thinking of us, giving to us, and I'm sure praying for us. I am continually astonished at where my encouragement comes from. Along with this, I received another card again today from Jerry's cousin Connie. We know from the

Bible that God is always with us. He constantly walks with us. And how does He do that? Through His people. I see it every day.

Thank you to all of you for everything you have done to encourage me.

Friday, October 10, 2008 1:17 a.m.

Hello dear friends,

It's been a busy few days. I've had busy classes and lots of meetings. I began the week tired, increased my energy during the week, and now am ending the week still a little tired. But that's okay. Being tired because of busyness is a good thing.

Many of you may know that I have been associated with Christian education my whole life. My parents chose to send me to Christian schools, we chose to send our children to Christian schools, and I've chosen to teach in Christian schools. Does that make me better than others who have not chosen Christian education? Certainly not. When I was growing up, people would sometimes call us the Post Toasties because they thought that we thought we were better than them. I'm afraid that sometimes we did portray that, and I'm sorry for that. Christian education is a choice parents make just as people choose public education, charter schools, magnet schools, etc. The choice I've made for Christian education doesn't make me a better person. This piece that follows I think does explain what it means to be a Christian. Carol Bootsma, a friend of mine, recently sent this to me. This piece was written by Maya Angelou, an African-American woman who advocates for peace among races.

"When I say . . . 'I am a Christian . . . '
   I'm not shouting 'I'm clean livin',' I'm whispering 'I was lost, now I'm found and forgiven.'
When I say . . . 'I'm a Christian'
   I don't speak with pride. I'm confessing that I stumble and need Christ to be my guide.
When I say . . . 'I'm a Christian'
   I'm not trying to be strong. I'm professing that I'm weak and need His strength to carry on.
When I say . . . 'I'm a Christian'
   I'm not bragging of success. I'm admitting I have failed and need God to clean my mess.
When I say . . . 'I'm a Christian'
   I'm not claiming I'm perfect, my flaws are far too visible but God believes I am worth it.

When I say . . . 'I'm a Christian'
>   I still feel the sting of pain . . . I have my share of heartaches, so
>   I call upon His name.
When I say . . . 'I'm a Christian'
>   I'm not holier than thou, I'm just a simple sinner who received
>   God's good grace, somehow!"

It is all about God's grace and I'm grateful He has chosen to lavish it upon me. If you are reading this, you've probably received His grace too. Praise the Lord! If not, please pray for His grace to come to you.

A bit about what's happening with me—my ears seem to have recovered. The burning pain has subsided. I'm still dealing with a dry forehead and cuts where my ears attach to my head but my right foot seems to be healing. I'm thankful for all the good things I'm experiencing.

Thanks again for your support.

Sunday, October 12, 2008 10:23 p.m.

Dear friends,

Over the weekend I received my beautiful quilt from Megan's friends in Michigan. What an awesome thing! What a humbling experience. And to think, Megan will have one just like it. When I look at the quilt, it will be a great reminder to pray for her, Mike, Amira and Nico, just as I will pray for Josh and Mindy, Sou, Kobi, Bailey and Miles.

I have to admit that after my diagnosis and the weeks following, I had a difficult time praying. It wasn't that I was angry, or maybe I was; I don't know, but I just couldn't pray. I've read about it, I've heard about it from others, but I don't think I've ever experienced it quite like this before. It's not that I even tried to pray. I just couldn't even think about it. Romans 8:26-27 says, "In the same way, the Spirit helps us in our weakness. We do not know what we ought to pray, but the Spirit himself intercedes for us with groans that words cannot express . . . the Spirit intercedes for the saints in accordance with God's will." Even when I didn't pray, when I couldn't pray, the Holy Spirit interceded for me, and He put it in the hearts of others to pray. I thank God for that promise and for you.

Just before my diagnosis, I was reading *Why Pray?* by John F. De Vries, the founder of a Christian non-profit organization called Mission India. In his book he talks about the amazing power of prayer. He relates story after story of how prayer turned lives around, how it provided for people, how it healed. I know that I have many prayer warriors out there. I don't know if God will heal me, but I do believe that God is very capable of taking away the cancer. Every day I thank God for people who are willing to pray for my healing.

I have about 36 days (who's counting) left before my MRI (Nov. 17). I'm thankful for work that keeps me too busy to worry too much. I'm thankful for prayers for peace and patience while I wait during this time. I'm thankful for modern medicine that can be used to heal.

I look forward to teaching about differentiation to my Ed. Psych students tomorrow. I'm thankful for my great students and the energy they give me. I'll need some extra energy as I cut down on the steroids this week, bringing me closer to the day I can be off them.

I hope you enjoy your week. Cella

Tuesday, October 14, 2008 8:53 a.m.

Good Morning,

A quick update, but first I want to say thanks for all your prayers! It is amazing how much they have lifted me up. My forehead has quit peeling; my ears have quit burning; and my right foot is looking much better. Dr. Krie suggested I put some anti-fungal ointment on it and it has really cleared up the redness. I am looking forward to today—I teach my largest and longest classes today. It takes much energy but I also receive much from it.

I am not sure if I shared this website with you. It tells about the mission of Carin and Carol Peters—www.margaretshopechest.com. If you scroll down to the bottom of the homepage (I think) you will see my quilt on the bottom of the pile. Isn't it beautiful? Have a good day.

Tuesday, October 14, 2008 11:09 p.m.

Hello dear friends,

Some of my colleagues accuse me of being able to play Dutch Bingo too well. Marion Van Soelen used to tell Kim S. and me that we knew more people than anyone else he knew. But I didn't realize that by referring to the website of those who gave me the quilt, a reader would get to play Dutch Bingo. Janie Van Dyke recognized the story behind the establishment of the quilt program and called to tell me that they are relatives of hers. Crazy isn't it? It seems we can find connections everywhere. Maybe it gets tiring for some to hear, "Ya, I know them!" but isn't that what life is all about? All of us are called to communities. That's what has kept me going the past two months. The support that we have experienced has given us strength and power to carry on. God wants us to live in community. He wants us to support others and accept support from others. It's a beautiful thing.

Some of you have probably read the story of Robinson Crusoe. It tells the story of an obstinate Englishman who ignored his father's wish for him to become a member of the clergy, opting instead for a life at sea. No sooner had his career started than he suffered a shipwreck and was cast ashore alive but alone somewhere on an uninhabited island off the coast of the New World. With only the supplies he salvaged from the wreck of his ship he managed to build a house, a boat and something of a life for himself. Despite living in a beautiful, idyllic location, Crusoe was never truly happy in his setting. The reason for his unhappiness was his solitude. It was not the climate, the food or setting that made him desperately unhappy. Rather, it was the fact that he was alone, "singled out and separated, as it were, from all the world, to be miserable." The island itself is not "a horrible, desolate island." It became horrible because of Crusoe's unbearable solitude. Community is a foundational part of God's design for humans.

The Bible, and the New Testament in particular, have many teachings on the importance of community. By studying two simple phrases that appear time and again in the New Testament, we can learn of the requirements and beauty of true Christian community. The phrases "each other" and "one another" speak to relationships.

Here are a few of the many passages that include the words "one another" or "each other."

"A new commandment I give you: Love one another. As I have loved you, so you must love one another. All men will know that you are my disciples if you love one another" (John 13:34-5, 1 Peter 1:22, 1 John 3:11).

"Be devoted to one another in brotherly love. Honor one another above yourselves" (Romans 12:10).

"Let no debt remain outstanding, except the continuing debt to love one another, for he who loves his fellow man has fulfilled the law" (Romans 13:8).

"Serve one another in love" (Galatians 5:13).

"Submit to one another out of reverence for Christ" (Ephesians 5:21).

We are thankful for the loving Christian community we live in.

Thursday, October 16, 2008 1:57 p.m.

Good Afternoon,

Just a quick update to let you know what is happening with me. I've experienced tremendous relief for my ears and head. My right foot is looking much better and feeling better too. Now I'm struggling a bit with energy. I've cut back on my steroids and am feeling the effect. The doctors told me this would happen, but I thought I could beat the odds. Not so. I was extremely tired yesterday, but I think I have more energy today. Yesterday was one of those days. After my class and meeting with a few students, I decided to miss our department meeting and go home to rest. I rested well and then planned for my class today. I had a great lecture written only to discover (late at night) that it somehow got deleted. Since it was late, I went to bed and hoped upon hope that the computer service people could find it for me this morning. Not so. It couldn't be found. So I spent some frantic moments reviewing the chapter and re-writing the lecture only to discover that I couldn't (for some reason) print it. So I went to class without notes. Thankfully we hadn't finished the last chapter so I finished that and then gave students a couple of reflective assignments that I believe were meaningful and we called it a day. I told the students that just as life doesn't always work out for them, it doesn't for us as instructors either. Another day in the life of a teacher. I love my job, even if it doesn't always go as I have planned.

Please continue to pray that my fatigue subsides and that the radiation is "doing its thing."

Thanks for your continued prayers, the food that keeps coming (just when I think I have to begin cooking, something shows up), the cards and notes of encouragement. In Him.

Sunday, October 19, 2008 11:14 p.m.

Dear friends,

I spent a good part of Saturday sleeping. Between naps I did the wash and worked on some school work. Friday night was late due to a reception that we had for parents following a long but beautiful concert. I took advantage of not having to be anywhere at a particular time on Saturday. We did meet my cousins, Bryan and Jill, for dinner in Orange City in the evening. It was nice to have a leisurely dinner and great conversation. After dinner Bryan took us to his place of employment which just happens to make the face mask and the table that were used for my radiation treatments. In fact, my mask had the brand name of his company right on the bottom of it. It was interesting to see the operation that actually manufactured the masks. I saw the flat masks and masks that looked like mine, indented and fit for the face. It's amazing for me to think of people actually coming up with and designing such things. But I am thankful that there are people out there who had a vision for designing equipment that helps apply the radiation. When I think of how far modern medicine has come in treating cancer, I am encouraged and thankful. God has provided us with many ways to fight this and other diseases.

I'm no theologian, but from what I understand, we don't see miracles today as they did years ago. Maybe it's because we have other means by which "miracles" happen. Dr. Brad Burke, author of *Does God Still Do Miracles?* says that we need to remember that miraculous healings may come in the forces that God already has in place. "God is definitely at work healing people today! If there's one thing I've learned in my journey as a physician, it's that God's ways are indeed higher than our own." He also says that whatever happens, as we ask for healing, we need to remember to trust God and rest in His perfect love for us. As I wait for my MRI on November 17, I will remember to trust God and rest in His love for me.

I'm ready for my classes tomorrow. I found the things I misplaced on Friday and already have my lecture ready for Tuesday. I hope I can find it all tomorrow.

I begin my last decrease in steroids tomorrow. That means taking the medication every other day for two weeks. I hope it doesn't take too long to adjust since I have long days at Dordt this week.

Thanks for your prayers, your encouragement through journal entries, notes, cards and personal conversations.

Wednesday, October 22, 2008 10:55 p.m.
Dear friends,

Today I came home early from school. I slept poorly last night due to a sore throat and congestion in my chest. I really considered not going in, but since I had only one class, I decided to get that in. I had two teeth filled yesterday; they were way back in my mouth and the cavities were deep, so I still have some pain in my mouth. We have a fantastic dentist in town, and I always appreciate his work, but it was difficult going into the appointment yesterday because his wife (my age) died within the last few weeks and I didn't know what I was going to say. It is always awkward to know what to say to someone who has just lost a loved one. But the conversation went well. We talked about the frailty of life and how quickly it can change. Tonight I went to the visitation of the father of two students I had at Dordt. He was killed in a construction accident earlier this week. Last week a cousin of mine from Sioux Falls (who is my age) died after suffering through cancer and then died of a stroke.

A classmate died because of cancer, and another woman I know is lying in the hospital with not much hope to live. All of these are reminders of how quickly our dreams, our hopes, our plans can change. I believe God wants us to make plans, but we always need to be aware that our plans will not always come to fruition. What we plan may be different from what happens. Even though I believe I can be cured of the cancer that has affected me, my case is a reality check for me. It does cause me to put my trust in God. Modern medicine is wonderful, but as my doctor said, "Only the [man upstairs] knows what is going to happen."

Being tired hasn't helped my attitude. It is harder to stay positive when my body hurts and has no energy. Please pray that I will soon have my energy back and that my cold symptoms will subside.

Thanks for all the cards I keep receiving. It amazes me how many of you continue to encourage me in this way. It is a great reminder that many are praying. In Him.

Friday, October 24, 2008 12:20 a.m.

Hello dear friends,

I hope I didn't sound too depressed in my last entry. Yesterday was my day to take the steroids so I felt a bit better. I don't know much about steroids so I don't know if they can change how you feel from day to day, but today it sure seemed as if they gave me a boost. I had a great lesson in my Foundation of Education class today. I wish all of you could experience the joy of teaching. I'm still coughing and sneezing some, but my sore throat is gone, and as I said, I do have more energy. The really good news is that my face is losing its puffy look. I actually have cheek bones again! For the last few weeks I've felt like a pumpkin with a nose. For someone who usually has a skinny face, this was not something I enjoyed looking at every morning when I looked in the mirror. While the fluid is draining from my face, there are other side effects that I will probably have to deal with for a while, one of them being weight gain. I never realized that steroids made one so hungry. I could eat a meal and sit right down and eat another one. Not a good idea! My appetite seems to be subsiding, but unfortunately, the weight hasn't fallen off yet. Something else to work on. Always things to work on, right?

In our Christian life, we are never complete and whole, are we. All of us are affected in some way by the sin that surrounds us. Thankfully we have a wonderful Heavenly Father who continues to work on us. I love the children's song "He Who Began a Good Work in You." It reminds us that "He will be faithful to complete it." It goes on to say, "If the struggle you're facing is slowly replacing your hope with despair, or the process is long and you're losing your song in the night, you can be sure that the Lord has His hand on you. Safe and secure He will never abandon you. You are His treasure and He finds His pleasure in you!"

I'm holding on to those promises!

Tuesday, October 28, 2008 9:12 p.m.

Dear friends,

It's been a few days since I wrote. I'm finding that coming off steroids is not as easy as going on them. I remember the day I came home from the hospital and wondered how I could feel so good and have so much energy. Well, steroids are the answer. I'm not sure if I'm right on this (correct me, nurses, if I'm wrong), but it seems that the days I take the steroids, I feel pretty good by noon and keep that feeling until evening. On my off days, I usually feel pretty draggy. On Saturday I'll take my last dose so we'll see what happens after that.

My department gave me a great gift today. They decided to do a group advising session in my freshman class so they told me I could have the day off. Thank you! It was great to have the day off, especially since it allowed me to take Jerry to the hospital for his scheduled carpal tunnel surgery. He wasn't supposed to drive home so it worked out well that I could go with him. His surgery went very well. Now he is walking around with his hand in the air and he's trying not to work. That's really difficult for him.

Jerry has been such a blessing to me through all my diagnoses and treatments that I was glad I could help him today. He has been patient, encouraging, always willing to serve, and always with a pleasant attitude. I often wonder if I would be that gracious and cheerful. I'm not sure. But I am very thankful for how he has stood by me. Who would have known that when we said our wedding vows and we promised to stick together through good times and bad, that it would lead to this. I'm thankful that Jerry has stood by me in the bad times. I hope we still can experience more good times. In Him.

Friday, October 31, 2008 11:50 p.m.

Dear friends,

Just when I begin to get nervous about what is happening in my brain, I get showered with unexpected blessings. Over the past few days, I've received cards from some very unexpected people. Such a blessing to know that many people care and pray. And then today I got a random e-mail from Megan. Wait, I need to back up. This morning when I opened my e-mail, I had a request from one of my cousins asking for Megan's phone number. I thought that was a bit strange but I e-mailed her Megan's number and told her some good times to reach her. I really wanted to ask her why, but I decided that if that information wasn't offered, it wasn't any of my business. Well, late this afternoon, Megan e-mailed me that someone called Judy De Wit had called her today. She didn't really know Judy so it took her a little while to figure out who this woman was. When she had it kind of figured out, Judy told her that my Vanden Bosch cousins had set up an account for her so that if she ever needed to come home, she would have some funds to make the trip. She, along with me, was astonished that anyone would do this for her.

When I thanked Judy for this wonderful display of love she related a few comments from family members. This is what a couple wrote: "So many people helped us with our daughters. I would be willing to give some money back. It's God's money—we just need to keep passing it around."

Judy ended her e-mail by saying, "And you are in all of the 'Vanden Bosch' cousins' prayers. Be assured of that. Colossians 4:2 says, 'Devote yourselves to prayer . . . . And then watch.'" That's what we're doing. Again, another humbling experience for all of us.

As Megan said, "Humbled. Awed. Inspired. Amazed! God is good . . . and His work through people and family is astounding."

We can never tell you how much we appreciate what all of you have done for us, whether it be words of encouragement, cards, gifts, prayers, whatever. You are a blessing.

Sunday, November 2, 2008 7:17 p.m.

Dear friends,

In Megan's thank-you e-mail to my relatives, she said, "I read an anonymous quote in our preparations to move to Nigeria that comes to mind as I once again reflect on God's faithfulness: 'I am carried on the shoulders of those who cannot see the landscape I describe. I owe them far more than my weight.' I am pretty sure I won't be able to repay fully all of you for the ways you are helping carry our family. But I do hope that in the future, far or near, that I will be in a position to give as you have given, remembering full-well the faithfulness of both our God and the Body of Believers when I do so."

Can you imagine not seeing the landscape and yet trusting that the person on your shoulder is telling you what he/she is seeing? Many of you are probably not experiencing my journey right now, and yet you are carrying us with your prayers and encouragement. Megan said, "In Nigeria we would say 'Mun Gode.' To you I say thank you. From the bottom of our hearts." That's what we say too!

Thank you from the bottom of our hearts! In Him.

Saturday, November 8, 2008 10:28 p.m.

Hello readers,

I imagine you were surprised to see the background on my site, weren't you. You would have probably expected to see something that matches what our landscape looks like now—snow. Well, I dislike snow and cold so much that I decided to brighten my day and put up a nice sunny day. I talked to Megan today and she said that it was 90 degrees at 6:00 in Nigeria. When I told her about our cold weather, she didn't think the 90 degree temperature sounded nearly so bad anymore. I camped out in the house today. It was too cold to go out and I had correcting to catch up on.

Even though I love teaching, it's nice to have the weekend to catch up on rest and on some extra school work. I've been off steroids for almost a week, but I'm still experiencing some fatigue. I hope that will improve over the next week. I can't believe I have just one more week before the MRI. I must say that I am a bit anxious, but your encouraging words have helped me focus on the big picture. (I continue to be amazed at the people who send cards.) I'd like to say that I have complete trust that God will heal me but in reality, I still have fears. Every time I cough or feel a new pain, I wonder if cancer is the cause. When I get a headache or wonder if my eyesight is fuzzy, I wonder if cancer could still be there. I hope that you will pray with me this coming week that I can stay calm, keep my eyes on God, and trust that He will do what is best for me. He promises that, you know. I just have to trust. Stay warm.

Monday, November 10, 2008 6:58 p.m.

Hello dear friends,

I'm usually not a worrier. I can usually take a deep breath and wait a bit before I get panicky. But when you are one week away from an MRI, funny things can happen to you. Over the past few days, I've wondered if my cough is something more than a cold. I've wondered if my runny nose is caused by trouble in my lungs. My back hurts sometimes and I've wondered if there could be something wrong with my bones. And then, over the past few days, I've been having difficulty with my eyesight.

Yesterday in church, I couldn't read the words in the song book very well, but it seemed I could read the numbers on the song board okay. Today as I drove to school, I felt as if I wasn't seeing as well as before. I wondered if the brain tumor was growing or maybe it had never disappeared. It is crazy what your thoughts can do to you. Well, when I got home, I decided to check to see if I had my contacts in the correct eyes. Sure enough, I had put my right contact in my left eye and my left contact in my right eye. I have mono-vision correction so one contact is stronger than the other. My brain, actually, makes it work. When I am looking at things in a distance, my right eye kicks in and vice versa. Well, that was the end of that problem. It taught me a few lessons, though: Don't read into things. Until I can't believe otherwise, I'll believe that the radiation did its job. As the Bible says, "Don't worry about tomorrow, because today has enough worries of its own."

I continue to feel humbled and thankful for your prayers and encouragement. Hope for warmer weather!

Thursday, November 13, 2008 12:16 a.m.

Dear friends,

I'd love to tell you that for the last few days I haven't felt anxious. I'd love to tell you that the knot in my stomach doesn't exist. I don't want to think about my eyes seeing correctly; yes, even with the correct contacts in my eyes. I wish I could say that every ache and pain that I'm experiencing doesn't have me worried about what is going on in my body; but if I did, I wouldn't be telling the truth. Even though I do trust that God will take care of me, I still have many worries and concerns. A lot of "what ifs." After next Monday I'll have some answers. I'll have a better picture of my future, at least for now. But until then I'm prone to worry. Please continue to pray with me that the tumor that remains will have shrunk and that no other tumors have grown. On Monday I'll be scheduling a PET scan for December. That will tell me if any cancer has reappeared in my body. I haven't been on any drugs since August so that is a concern too.

God has been good through this whole ordeal. He has given me all of you! Thanks much for all your encouragement. It has come in many ways. Each day I am amazed by the people who either call, send a card, or give some kind of personal encouragement.

In Romans 15:30, Paul says, "I urge you, brothers, by our Lord Jesus Christ and by the love of the Spirit, to join me in my struggle by praying to God for me." Please join me in my struggle. Thank you.

Thursday, November 13, 2008 10:33 p.m.

Dear friends,

Last Sunday evening Catherine Schreur and I played for Mindy's special music at Hull Hope CRC. (Sherri, I said yes to this before I got your e-mail.) Cath played the viola and I played the piano. I love playing with Cath. She is very accomplished and everyone loves to listen to her as she plays the melody, so I feel no pressure as I play the accompaniment. The song we chose was a medley that went through many of the themes of the Bible. We've played this song before and we always say that it begins Christian Reformed and ends Baptist! We love this song and so do many others. People can't seem to hold their heads still when we end with "There is Power in the Blood." The title of the medley is "The Music of God's Family." Along with many other very recognizable songs throughout the medley, the first and last part of the song reminds us that we are all part of God's family. And that is what I have truly experienced over the past two years. I always knew there were many caring people out there, but there is nothing like experiencing it firsthand, even though it is because of illness.

In Pastor Todd's sermon on Sunday night, he talked about being thankful, yes, in all circumstances. Paul doesn't tell us to be thankful for everything. The footnote to I Thessalonians 5:18 in the NIV Bible says, "Evil does not come from God, so we should not thank him for it. But when evil strikes, we can still be thankful for God's presence and for the good that He will accomplish through the distress." Even though I would have preferred not to have to go through this experience, I have to admit that once again I was shown the power of God's people. This week I've received phone calls from those I don't know well; cards from people I've never met; and hugs from close friends. Some I don't know, some I know a little, and some I know well. Amazing isn't it?

Thank you from the bottom of my heart for all the ways you support me.

Monday, November 17, 2008 12:34 a.m.

Dear praying friends,

Well, here we are—D-day! In some ways I thought it would never get here and yet in some ways, I'm surprised it is here already. In any case, I'm glad we've reached the day. You have all been a great blessing to me. During the weekend I received many well-wishes. I continue to pray for a good report, but I also try to be realistic in my thoughts. I'm very aware that the report can go either way, but I also know that no matter what happens, God will be there. This weekend my friend Linda sent me a great cartoon. I tried to copy it in this site, but it wouldn't take it. Since I couldn't add it, I'll give you a verbal description. Here is my attempt:

On the bottom of the picture was this text: "Look at the birds of the air; they do not sow or reap or store away in barns, and yet your Heavenly Father feeds them. Are you not much more valuable than they? Who of you by worrying can add a single hour to his life?" (Matthew 6:26-27). Above it was a picture of a man with his head in his hands. Around him were words like stress, anxieties, worries, debt, and bills. There were two birds sitting in the open window sill. One said to the other, "What's eatin' him?" "I don't know," the other one said. "I guess God doesn't take care of him like He does us." That says it all, doesn't it? If God cares for the birds, how much more does He care for us, his people.

Thanks again for your prayers. You've been a part of this whole process and we couldn't appreciate you more. I'll write on the CaringBridge site as soon as I can to let you know what the MRI read. My MRI is scheduled for 10:30 and then I'll have it read at 3:30 by Dr. Krie so it will be sometime after that.

Please continue to pray boldly and humbly for good news. In Him.

Monday, November 17, 2008 5:07 p.m.

Hello everyone,

I wanted to write a quick update (mom will write more later). I talked to mom a little while ago and her appointment went well today. The spot in the front shows a little residue, but they think that is left from the surgery and shows no sign for concern and the tumor in the back shrunk from 22 mm to 7 mm. That is amazing and the best news that we could have asked for today. They aren't planning any treatments right now because the radiation could still be working. Thank you all for your thoughts and prayers; we have definitely felt them! Mindy

Tuesday, November 18, 2008 6:22 a.m.

Dear friends,

First of all, thank you much for your prayers. God does miraculous things through His people. I was extremely anxious the past few weeks with each day causing me more anxiety. I was sure I had more pressure on my right eye. I wasn't so sure my vision was what it should be. That, plus aches and pains in my body, all led to some very anxious thoughts. I've had a pain in the pit of my stomach for days. So when Dr. Krie told us good news, we were almost too astonished to respond. It wasn't that we doubted God; we knew He could use the radiation to shrink the tumor, but would it happen? We thank God for His healing mercies, and we pray they will continue. The radiation could work up to two more weeks. I'll have another MRI in two to three months to see what is happening. I'm scheduled for a PET scan the end of December to see what is going on in my body. We feel very grateful for this good news—we are humbly rejoicing in the healing that has taken place.

All we can say now is, Praise God from whom all blessings flow! In Him.

Wednesday, November 19, 2008 9:44 p.m.

Dear friends,

A friend Abbie Van Essen sent me this e-mail yesterday and it really reminded me of my life. It reminded me of the leanin' I've been doing the past few months. I'm sure many of you can relate to it too, so I'm going to share it with you. Here it is:

> Every time I am asked to pray, I am reminded of the old deacon who always prayed, Lord, prop us up on our leanin' side. After hearing him pray that prayer many times, I asked him why he prayed that prayer so fervently.
>
> He answered, "Well sir, you see it is like this—got an old barn out back. It's been there a long time. It's withstood a lot of weather; it's gone through a lot of storms; and it's stood for many years. In fact, it's still standing. But one day I noticed that it was leaning to one side a bit. So I went and got some pine poles and propped them up against the leaning side so it wouldn't fall."

Then I got to thinking about that and how much I was like that old barn. I've been around a long time too; I've withstood many storms; I've withstood a lot of bad weather in life; I've withstood a lot of hard times, but I'm standing too. But I find myself leaning to one side from time to time, so I like to ask the Lord to prop me up on my leanin' side. I figure we all get to leanin' at times.

Sometimes we get to leanin' toward anger, sometimes toward bitterness, other times toward lack of trust, other times leaning toward cussing', leanin' toward a lot of things we shouldn't do. So we need to pray, "Lord, prop us up on our leanin' side, so we will stand straight and tall again, so we can glorify God."

I'm thankful for the support I had while I "leaned" the past few months. What would I have done without your support?

I'm finding that my anxiety is lessening as I get past the MRI. I had a difficult time believing the MRI—that the tumor had truly decreased. I had a difficult time grasping the good news. I didn't want to be pessimistic, but I also wanted to be realistic. I didn't want to be so overconfident that I would be crushed if the radiation hadn't worked. When Dr. Krie told me the news, I think she was surprised by my reaction. (Am I right, Dr. Krie?) I was quite stunned and didn't really know how to react. I must admit, I was ready for less encouraging news. I may face other issues in the future, but for now I can enjoy the holiday season. I've told myself to stop looking for signs of cancer. But I guess even though I'm thrilled by the reading of the MRI, I will probably continue to slip back into doubt and fear occasionally; that's when I'll go to leanin' on the Giver of Life. And even when I lean, I hope I can still continue to glorify God. I hope, if you need it, you can find the poles to lean on too.

Thanks for your support.

Thursday, November 20, 2008 10:04 p.m.

Dear friends,

I'm sitting here tonight wrapped in a blanket, listening to the fire as it crackles in the fireplace. I love to hear the sound of the wood popping and watch the flames as they dance in the metal grate. The firecracker-like sparks shoot up as the wood breaks apart, giving the fireplace an orange glow. Jerry does a great job of building a fire. A fire gives warmth and a cozy feeling.

A number of years ago, when our daughters were still in high school, we were sitting in the living room one evening with a fire like the one I'm enjoying tonight. I remember— it was Jerry, Mindy, Megan, her friend Laura, and me. While I watched everyone practice their head stands (Jerry was the best), talk, and laugh, I commented, "Isn't this romantic." They all burst out laughing. They didn't think the situation merited being called romantic. I don't know why. I miss that laughter that was such a big part of our home as the kids grew up. I miss the action that took place in our living room as we gathered around the fireplace to go over the activities of the day.

What a blessing to have good family memories! I'm thankful that we can remember the fun we've had together over the years. We still laugh about the time Jerry took us all through the median at DisneyWorld. Sou and Mike had never been on a ride like that before! Then there's the time Megan and Mindy (accidentally) started the house on fire and if it hadn't been for the fast-acting firemen, we would have lost our house. I could probably write a host of other "memories" but I don't want to bore you. My point is that even though we've experienced some hard times, we are very grateful for all the fun times we have had as a family.

I Thessalonians 5:16 says, "Be joyful always; . . . ." We are glad for the times our family has been able to laugh and do crazy things together. We also joy in the times we've experienced hardships and sadness. We know that true joy doesn't come from circumstances and things, but in the hope we receive from the promises of our Lord. I hope you also experience that true joy that can only come from God.

We continue to be blessed with your cards, words, and hugs. Thank you.

Tuesday, November 25, 2008 6:58 p.m.

Dear friends,

Have you wondered where I've been the past few days? On the couch, literally! Ever since the weekend I've really struggled with fatigue and nausea. If I ate, I felt sick and if I didn't eat, I felt sick. Sad thing was, I didn't lose any weight even when I didn't eat. Jerry made me promise to call Dr. Krie to see what was up. Dutifully I did, and she said it sounded like my symptoms were the result of going off the steroids too quickly. So, that means back to steroids. I took two pills this morning and I don't know if it is coincidental or what, but I did feel better today. I had a lot more energy (didn't take a nap all day) and I even ate a bit and didn't feel or get sick. Now I hope I can sleep tonight! It was disappointing to have to go back on steroids, but I knew I couldn't live as I was. I first attributed my fatigue to a busy weekend—an education department retreat in Sioux Falls on Friday and Saturday morning, a movie with my grandsons in the afternoon, church on Sunday morning and then a Thanksgiving dinner with my family at my sister's house. But how much can a person sleep? Twelve hours seems a bit excessive!

Thanksgiving—it's just around the corner. It's a wonderful time of year! It's a great time to spend with family and friends. Some of you may share delicious meals with those you love. You may also hunt, shop, get out your Christmas decorations, or whatever you love to do. But in all the excitement of celebrating, I hope you take time to thank God genuinely for all the blessings He has showered on you. In Dr. Zylstra's chapel address yesterday he said, "The spirit of Thanksgiving does not really have to depend on whether or not a year is particularly prosperous or filled with delightful occurrences. The Lord remains our Sovereign God and Gracious Savior in all circumstances." It's something I need to continue to remember as I face issues with cancer. It's as Pastor Todd said in his sermon a few Sunday nights ago, "Be joyful always; pray continually; give thanks in all circumstances, for this is God's will for you in Christ Jesus" (I Thessalonians 5:16-18). I'm thankful for God's presence in my life. I hope you are too.

Have a blessed Thanksgiving!

Wednesday, November 26, 2008 11:56 a.m.

A quick update on how I'm feeling—I didn't go to sleep until after 10:00 last night and this morning I cleaned three cupboards and cleaned some spots out of the carpet. Do you think the steroids are working? I can't believe how quickly the pills have changed how I feel. They must be pretty powerful, huh? I'm thankful for the wisdom of doctors and pills they can prescribe.

Thursday, November 27, 2008 8:08 a.m.

Good Morning,

Have a Blessed Thanksgiving. What a beautiful day even in Northwest Iowa. But even if the sun wasn't shining, it would be a wonderful day. It's a day set aside as an American holiday for us to give thanks for all the blessings each one of us has received during the past year and beyond. I'm sure all of you who are reading this can think of oodles of things for which you are thankful. For some it may be material blessings but that might not be the case for everyone. All of us can thank God for the way He has walked in our life in the past year. I'm thankful for the way God has carried us through the past year. I'm thankful for the wisdom of doctors, for researchers who have developed new medicines, for medical technicians and nurses who pleasantly minister to my needs. I'm also thankful for all of you and for the many ways you have supported us. You have truly exemplified Christ, whether it be through prayer, rides, notes of encouragement, encouraging conversations, food, monetary gifts, etc. Thank you.

Listen to these Old Testament words (something written long before this holiday was established): "Give thanks to the LORD, call on his name; make known among the nations what he has done, Sing to him, sing praise to him; tell of all his wonderful acts . . . . Look to the LORD and his strength; seek his face always" (I Chronicles 16:8-9, 11).

We love you all and wish you a wonderful Thanksgiving with family and friends. In Him, Jerry and Cella

Sunday, December 7, 2008 11:35 p.m.

Hello friends,

I can't believe how much time has passed since the last time I wrote in my journal. Jerry just reminded me that I haven't posted anything for over a week. Must be good to be busy, right?

I've felt good the past week. Going back on steroids was a good thing for me. I'm now taking them every other day and that seems to be working. I have a very busy week, not so much in teaching but in grading, so I hope my energy keeps up enough to finish the semester well. I was going to work very hard at not having so much correcting at the end of the semester, but my freshman classes seem to need as much time learning in class before I can ask them to complete a few assignments, so once again I've "worked" my way into a lot of grading at the end of the semester.

On Saturday I went with Nate, Catherine, and Chyann to Kanawha. I go there once a year on the first Saturday in December to play with Cath at the community brunch that the Christian Reformed Church provides for the community. It is always a beautiful event. Each table is decorated by a hostess. It's amazing how each table was "Christmasy" and yet unique, bringing out the character of each hostess.

Every other year Cath and I have been the "entertainment." Cath plays the viola and I play the piano. We love being able to play the Christmas music that we really get to play in only one month during the year. This year, instead of just playing, I was also asked to speak. It surprised me that I would get so nervous. I'm used to talking in front of some pretty good-sized classes, but this speech was in front of well over 125 women and it was about me. I'm not wild about talking about myself so deciding what to say was difficult. I didn't want the speech to be a woe-is-me kind of speech, and yet I knew they asked me to speak because of my story. I decided to take the idea of David Smith and talk about being in the garden. As I did some research and then wrote, I realized how much it was my attitude that determined my Garden of Delight. Sometimes I really wish that I could just wipe the past two years out of my life. I wish I didn't have to continue to worry about cancer returning or if it has returned. I wish I didn't have to worry about the side effects of the medication. But I do. And that is part of my life right now. And just as I mentioned earlier, it is my choice of how I am going to deal with it. I can be anxious, sad, angry, or have a host of other negative feelings. Or I can look for the many ways that God has blessed and continues to bless me, even through cancer. I can praise God for all my prayer warriors; I can praise Him for all the encouragement I've received and continue to receive from family, friends, and even those I don't know personally. I can praise God for the great medical profession and all the technology that has aided in my healing. And I do thank and praise God each day for His wonderful care that I'm experiencing through His people. Of course, this isn't done on my own. I thank God for giving me the ability to see the Garden of Delight even amongst hardships. Each of you has probably experienced some trial or tribulation in your life too. Trials and tribulations aren't what cause us to be unable to find our Garden of Delight. It's our attitude. When we look for the delight, we can find it. I hope you see your Garden of Delight as you work and play this week. Thanks for your prayers.

Have a good week.

Wednesday, December 10, 2008 12:02 a.m.

Hello dear praying friends,

This is the part of having to drive to Sioux Center that I dread—icy and snowy roads. Just think, we haven't even technically gotten to winter and already we are having late starts and cancellations. Winter looks like a long season when it begins so early. I'm sure all my teacher friends were eagerly listening for a late start, but I'm sure no one was hoping for a cancellation. Having snow days before Christmas is something teachers don't want. I don't get the "joy" of listening to the radio or TV to check for late starts or a cancellation of school any more. Now don't get me wrong, it's not that I didn't love to teach when I was in elementary school, but there was always this element of anticipation—what was going to happen? Since school at Dordt goes on no matter what the weather, I prepared for Jessica to help me with my classes today, just in case I couldn't make it in. Even though the roads were a little snowy, driving on them wasn't bad at all. Of course, some drivers thought the roads were worse than I did, but all in all it wasn't bad driving in. I usually take the Highway 60 bypass and then B40 but when the roads have the potential for being slippery, I stick to the main highways. As I drove this morning I thought about all the safe travel I have had over the years. Not only have I driven back and forth to Dordt safely, but I've also driven the busy truck route in New Mexico, the hilly areas of Minnesota, and the flat roadways of Iowa, all safely. I'm thankful for all that safety.

Although I've been safe on the roads, the sidewalks have been a different story for me. While at Dordt, I've tripped on a lip on the sidewalk and ripped open my knee. I've caught my toe on a piece of plywood that was serving as a sidewalk and sprawled right onto the lawn, and then a few years ago I slipped on the ice in the parking lot and jammed my hand into the curb. How did I do that? I don't know; some things just happen that I can't explain. The doctor called my break a barroom brawl break. He said that the kind of break I had is usually a result of a barroom brawl. Believe me, I wasn't in a bar and I surely didn't smack anybody. My slip today wasn't anything like that. I was very carefully treading my way to my car. I was wearing very flat snow boots (no high heels for me) and moving slowly on the icy sidewalks and just lost my footing. Kyle was walking beside me and before he knew it, I was down on the ground. It happened so fast neither of us knew how it happened. I was, of course, drinking a Diet Coke which went flying into the snow. With the help of Kyle and Paul, I got up and they guided me to my car. Now besides suffering from steroid withdrawal and muscle pain, I have new pains resulting from the fall. My poor right hip always seems to get the short-end of the deal. It could be a long winter!

Our semester is almost over. I have just three classes left to teach. But I'm not quite finished. I have about 75 philosophy statements, 75 educational philosophy brochures and papers, and 75 tests to grade. I'm not complaining. Assessment comes with the job. I love to see what the students have learned, but staying unbiased and consistent is always difficult. How do I treat each student as a unique creation of God and yet hold them to certain standards? How do I encourage the students and bring out their strengths and build on their weaknesses? Those are hard questions for me to answer, and I'm afraid I haven't figured it out very well yet.

Today I handed out evaluations for Education 101. Each semester the students evaluate each class to help us improve our teaching. Wouldn't it be something if we could receive feedback about our life? The Bible gives us guidelines, and from there we have to do our own evaluating. Do we? Do we do a self-check based on what Jesus taught us in the gospels? Do we look at what Paul teaches us and match our life to his instructions? Or is it easier to read what they say and then keep on doing what we are doing? I'm afraid I find myself doing that more than I should. I'm going to be taking a good look at the gospels during the next few weeks and work on evaluating my spiritual life. What a good time of year to do a self-evaluation. Thanks for all your prayers and support. I continue to feel your love and care. Even amidst the cold, snowy weather, I hope you have a good week. In Him.

Thursday, December 11, 2008 12:23 a.m.

Dear friends,

A few weeks ago my cousin Lynnette was watching her niece Skyler when she fell hard and put a hole in her knee. She had to go to the doctor to have four stitches to "fix it up." When she left for the doctor, this is how Lynnette described her: "When she headed to the doctor she reminded me of Mindy as a little girl. She had on one orange sock, one striped sock, a nice purple top, and a lime green skirt which was really a sundress that she now wears as a skirt because it's way too small. She did not originally look this unkempt, but we did not want to put the purple pants on again. She was responsible for packing the mismatched socks and came to my house the day before in the dress worn as a skirt. "Tell me this outfit does not remind you of Mindy as a youngster." She was so right. When Mindy was little, we would tell her she had to change her clothes before she could come along with us uptown. She too would put on the oddest combinations—gaudy, flamboyant, showy. (Sounds a little like Amira's choices, huh, Megan?) The other day Amira put on the cutest little outfit. It was a blue gingham top with matching blue capris. Megan was quite amazed because usually she couldn't get Amira to wear this rather trendy outfit. Well, to no surprise, after she ate breakfast Amira went back to her room and put on the "rest" of her outfit—multi-striped knee highs and pink cowboy boots. She made quite a fashion statement! She was very comfortable with how she was dressed, just as Skyler and Mindy were comfortable with how they dressed.

It seems that sometimes we concentrate so much on the outside that we neglect the inside. Mindy, Skyler, and Amira didn't worry about what others thought of how they looked on the outside. (I'm not sure they were that concerned at that point how they looked on the inside either, but it does say that they were very comfortable with who they were.) They didn't feel as if they had to impress anyone. Are we like that or are there times when we are more concerned with our outward appearance rather than our inside appearance?

God tells us in I Samuel 16:7 that He looks at the heart of a person and not at what a person looks like on the outside. When we judge by outward appearances, we can overlook quality people who lack the physical appearances that our culture today tells us are important. In one of the classes I teach, we talk about "lookism." It's a term that refers to who gets hired for a job, to how we respond to new people who walk into our church, to how we talk to an employee at a fast-food restaurant. How do we respond to those around us? What do we look at? I must say, I've been guilty of looking on the outside as I "size up" people. I'm quite sure that isn't what God wants me to do. As I move about the community during this holiday season, I hope my eyes will be "blind" to the outward appearance of those with whom I come into contact and instead concentrate on seeing their inner beauty.

Even though it's a busy season, it's a blessing to have this time to remember many who mean much to us. I hope you all enjoy your family and friends.

I love the children's song "What Can I Give Him?" It is a good reminder that each of us must remember to give God our heart. I wonder how you would describe the giving of your heart. Joy for the day.

P.S. By the way, I survived my fall but I did encourage the maintenance department to spread a little salt.

Saturday, December 13, 2008 1:30 a.m.

Dear friends,

Maybe I shouldn't have gone. I don't know if I was ready for it. All the way home I was on the verge of tears but instead of crying, I bottled them up and acted as if nothing was wrong. We kidded about my driving on the way to Sioux Center, but we didn't discuss the issue. Just for a little background, we once again left late from home to attend the 10:00 p.m. play at the New World Theatre. We stopped to see a friend in the hospital and then at McDonald's for Jerry to get some take-out. Well, just in case you need to know this, the Sheldon McDonald's is not fast food. It took Jerry forever to get his food. By that time I was quite irritated so I decided it would be much to our advantage for me to drive. Those of you who know me well, know what that means. The stage manager, also a student of mine, was saving us seats but could only save them until 20 minutes before show time. I didn't want to drive all the way to Sioux Center at that time of night and then not be able to get in. Half the cast have been or are now my students so I really wanted to see them in action. With my expert driving, we made it on time.

I knew the content of the play; I knew it dealt with cancer, and I knew it dealt with dying. But I didn't know it would be so real. I didn't know that Jenna would act her part superbly, and I didn't know it would bother me. But it did. When Jenna yelled, "I'm scared," I thought, "Yah, I'm scared too." I don't like wondering what is happening in my body. I don't like wondering about the future. I know, we've talked about living for today; we all know that anyone could die at any time, but death does seem much more real to me now that I'm dealing with cancer.

Sometimes I am scared. I think about the future and I wonder how much of it I will see. And yet I have the confidence, not on my own, but with God's grace, that He will carry me through. He promises this and I have to believe it. I'm comforted by the Advent words, "I know that my Redeemer lives, and that He shall stand at the latter day upon the earth: And though worms destroy this body, yet in my flesh shall I see God" (based on Job 19:25-26).

It reminds me of the first question and answer from the Heidelberg Catechism: "What is your only comfort in life and in death? That I am not my own, but belong—body and soul, in life and in death—to my faithful Savior, Jesus Christ." I'm thankful for that. I hope you are too.

Thanks for the many ways you continue to encourage us. In Him.

Sunday, December 14, 2008 10:12 p.m.

Dear faithful readers,

As I'm sure you've all noticed, I changed the design of my website. It was time to let go of summer and the beach and become season appropriate. I chose the gift design because of the season. God's gift to us is the best thing any of us could ever receive. In turn, we take time during this season to give gifts to others.

A good friend of mine (Linda) sent me this reflection on life. It seemed to fit so well with the Garden of Delight that I mentioned last week that I wanted to share it with you too.

Nothing happens by accident. If one day when you woke up, you would find on your bed a beautifully wrapped present with delicate bows, you would open it before even washing your face, curious about what's inside. Maybe what you would find is something you do not like very much, and you would put it away, wondering what to do with it. But if the next day you would find another present, open it, and this time you found something inside that you liked very much:
- a memory from someone who is far away
- a gorgeous coat which you saw in a shop window
- a beautiful flower from someone who remembered you.

How would you react? This happens every day but we do not always realize it. Every day when we wake up, it is there, before us, a present sent to us from God, a whole day to use in the best way possible. Sometimes it comes with problems, issues that we do not seem to be able to solve. Sometimes it comes with sadness, even tears. But other times it comes full of surprises, happiness, success, and achievement.

What is important is that every day we receive a present wrapped especially for us while we sleep: THE NEXT DAY. We are presented this box with colored bows, no matter what the day brings. Every morning is a present. Inside the present is the life we've been given. It is not always what we wish for or what we hope for, but it is the best for us, what we need most, what we have to learn, what we need to grow.

Open your present every day, giving thanks first to the Creator who gave it to you, without thinking what is inside the box. If today you did not receive the present you wanted, wait for the next one, and appreciate what you received today.

May you have a day full of blessings in which you can feel the loving presence of our Creator, and may the "present" of every day bring you peace, spiritual growth, lessons to learn about each day, and the plans God has for you today.

I took my last dose of steroids today. I felt myself getting more tired as the week progressed, but I hope with fewer demands on my time this week, I'll be able to handle the fatigue and begin to gain back some energy. I have much correcting to do this week; I hope I'll be able to focus and persevere through the task. Stay warm.

Tuesday, December 23, 2008 12:29 p.m.

Dear friends,

As you may have noticed, Mindy changed the picture on the front page. We do have a tradition of going out each Thanksgiving Day afternoon and cutting a tree from a tree farm. The past few years we have had to bundle up because of the frigid temperatures. This year was no different! It was cold but we at least didn't have to tromp through any snow. As Jill said, yes, we usually have a good story to tell with our annual tree-cutting but this year was quite uneventful. The best story was probably the year that Jerry had his toe surgery and was taking quite a heavy dose of pain killers (at least that's what we blame it on). He couldn't get out of the vehicle to check for a straight trunk so we, of course, found a beautiful tree but you guessed it, a crooked trunk. Jerry was insistent that we keep cutting the trunk in order to straighten it out and get it to stand in the tree stand. By the time we finished, it was a pretty short tree. We ended up calling it our "Sou tree." Those of you who know Sou will know the "rest of the story."

The tradition of celebrating Christmas has gone on for a couple thousand years now. While that tradition goes on, we've developed some of our own family traditions. As you read above, selecting and cutting our trees has become one of our family traditions. We've missed Michael, Megan, Amira, and Nico the past couple of years. (Oh, just to let you know, those scraggly pine branches in the picture were not our Christmas trees.) We've also developed the tradition of dressing up in our warmest clothes and heading out on Christmas Eve to sing Christmas carols for special people in our lives. For me there is nothing better than seeing the smiles on people's faces as we sing in our "Bosma" key. No one cares that we can't all keep perfect pitch. No one cares if some of us forget a few of the words and have to hum through those parts. But everyone seems to enjoy seeing familiar faces sing familiar songs of great joy.

Caroling on Christmas Eve is a very small gift that we give to others. It doesn't cost us anything, proving that gifts don't have to cost money. Sometimes our presence, our time, our attention are the best things we can give. Today I believe I received the best present I will get this Christmas. It didn't cost money but it did take some time. One of my students, Jonathan Brue, whom I taught last semester, sent me an e-mail thanking me for my teaching this past semester. I cried as I read the e-mail (and even as I write this I can feel the tears running down my cheeks). I'm sure he'll never know how much his note meant to me. The past semester was difficult. It's a good thing I love teaching, because it pretty much consumed my life. But as I taught I wondered if I was being effective. I wondered, "Are the students really learning from me?" "Am I teaching them what it is going to take to become an effective teacher?" I'm not sure I was effective with all my students, but I must have touched this particular student. His words will forever stay with me. It was a great reminder for me to thank people in my life for the wonderful things they have done for me. It doesn't take an expensive gift to say "thanks"; words of appreciation are really the best gift any of us can give. I hope you too can thank someone personally for a "gift" they have given to you. Maybe it's a past teacher, minister, youth leader, coworker, coffee partner, or friend.

I love all of you and wish I could personally say thanks for the encouragement you have given to me over the past couple of years, but since I can't, please consider this as personal as it will get: "THANKS." Thanks for your prayers and for all the other acts of kindness. We couldn't have done it without you.

Have a Blessed Christmas as you spend time with family and friends, celebrating the greatest GIFT we received through the birth of Jesus Christ.

Please continue to pray that I get over the hump from the effects of taking the steroids. I'm really struggling with fatigue and very sore muscles, plus a right foot that is acting up again. Love.

Thursday, December 25, 2008 10:35 a.m.
Merry Christmas!

For to us a child is born, to us a son is given,
and the government will be on his shoulders.
And he will be called Wonderful Counselor, Mighty God,
Everlasting Father, Prince of Peace. (Isaiah 9:6)

What a comfort to know that the Prince of Peace came to bring me (us) peace, not an earthly peace but an everlasting peace. I wish you all a very blessed day as you worship God with your family and friends in your celebrations. Merry Christmas.

Sunday, December 28, 2008 12:16 a.m.
Slowly sliding through the MRI machine, I reflected on the events of the past few days.

Sore muscles, shooting pain, a right foot that felt frozen or like a club foot, numb buttocks cheeks, an incredibly tender bottom of my left foot, a draggy right leg, weakness when climbing stairs.

Those were the symptoms that prompted me to call Dr. Krie on Friday morning. I called because I wanted some medication for the neuropathy I had self-diagnosed for myself. When she didn't call back by 5:15, I decided I should call once more to make sure she would get the call for the prescription into the pharmacy before the store closed. This time I connected with Dr. Krie; she asked a few questions and then said she didn't feel comfortable ordering medication with the symptoms she was hearing. She requested that we head to Sioux Falls, check into the ER and have an MRI. That didn't bother me too much. I knew that I needed medication to lessen the pain I was having and if that's what I needed to do, I was willing to do it.

So we headed out in the dense fog. Thankfully it was evening by the time we left Sanborn so visibility was helped with the contrast of headlights and darkness. Jerry was a little tense as we drove. At one point he pushed his back against the driver's seat and said, "What am I doing, leaning over the steering wheel like this? I can see just as good if I sit back." That did help him relax.

We arrived at a very busy ER, waited our turn, and then were placed in an exam room. After what seemed like ages, the technician from the

MRI room came and took me for the scan. I found out I am getting pretty good at tolerating the noise of the machine. I also discovered that the pain medication they had given me wasn't touching my pain, so for the last half hour, I had to resist pinching that little ball that tells the scanners, "HELP! I need to get out right now!"

Then the wait. Honestly, we were not nervous. Jerry and I were pretty confident that all I needed was medication to help calm down the neuropathy. When the ER doctor came in and told us that it was cancerous tumors that were causing the pain and numbness, we were stunned. It was not the news we were expecting. After adjusting to the news, we moved to a room on the oncology floor and tried to settle in for the night.

This morning an oncologist/radiologist came in to explain a bit more. He said that just as the brain has a protective zone, so does the spinal cord. Just as the brain isn't affected by chemo, so it is with the spinal cord. (At least that is what we understood him to say. With so much new information, we are constantly wondering if we are hearing information correctly.) But it does respond to radiation, just like the brain. So they immediately set up a time for me to begin radiation. Before treatments could begin, I had to be measured and a "plan" had to be drawn that was just for my disease. The setup took a bit of time, but the treatment, just as with the radiation to the brain, took just a few minutes.

So the sad news for us was the diagnosis of cancer in yet another spot, but the good news of the day is that the MRI which they took of my brain later this morning showed no active cancer cells.

If you are reading this and you are over fifty, I think you can relate to my fear as I awaited the results of the brain MRI. Have I been losing words because of my age or something more serious? Am I losing my train of thought because of my age or is cancer in the brain causing this? Am I losing strength because of "old age" or something more serious? Why do I feel pain where I've never felt pain before? Why can't I bend like last year? (Last year I bent like a piece of licorice and this year I feel like a toothpick.) And so much more. So it was with great relief to hear that my symptoms are, at this point, just "old age." I never thought I'd be glad to hear that my body is falling apart because of my age, but I rejoiced today.

I'm not sure what is going to happen over the next few days, but I will keep you posted. We are very confident that the treatments will be as successful as were the brain radiation treatments. Dr. Krie feels that for now, I should be able to go on with life just as I did with the brain radiation.

Once again we are asking you to join us on yet one more hill on the roller coaster ride, the journey of life. We ask that you help us in praying for positive results from the treatments. Thanks for allowing us to join your prayer list.

In Him, Jerry and Cella

Monday, December 29, 2008 12:14 a.m.

To my prayer warriors,

Mystery—that's a word that keeps coming back to me as I reflect on the happenings of the past few days or I guess I could say, the past few years. But then again, maybe my whole life. My life, like yours, is a mystery and that mystery is something that won't end until we reach eternity. Some of the mysteries I've lived through were best left mysteries, unfolding slowly, giving me time to "grow" into the situation. I think of Josh's accident and its results; I think of my hip surgery and its strange events. And now I think of my cancer. It has been and continues to be a mystery to me. The mystery lies in the questions. Will it come back? If so, where will it show up? Will the doctors be able to continue to find medication that can stop the cells from spreading? Rob Bell says that the "Christian faith is mysterious to the core. It is about things and beings that ultimately can't be put into words. Language fails. And if we definitively put God into words, we have at that very moment made God something God is not."

A mystery happens when we can't see key facts, when we can't see the end. So that is how it is for me. I can know about the cancer that I have now, but where will it end? Will the doctors find a treatment that can control the cells? So far they have, but what will happen in the future is unknown. It is a mystery.

But because of these mysteries, I have found myself looking more intensely at God, trying to understand who He is, how He loves me, why He loves me, what He wants me to do, and on and on and on. In chapters 38 to 41 God reminds Job of His power and wisdom which is beyond the capacity of Job. A mystery! I feel like Job who ended up saying,"God is just too big for me." As my life unfolds, I am learning more about God—about His endless love, about the ways He leads me to get to know Him better.

Mysteries in books end in the last chapter. Mysteries are meant to be solved. The mystery of life will end too—when we get to heaven. Until then, I hope to keep living and, to the best of my ability, to serve God.

The mystery I have for now is: Where will we go from here? Tomorrow Dr. Krie and I will discuss the next move we make. It looks like I will get dismissed from the hospital in Sioux Falls on Tuesday, have my PET scan on Wednesday a.m., and a consultation with Dr. Krie in the afternoon. There are many unknowns right now. I hope after the PET scan we will know more. I'll let you know more as I find out more.

Thanks for your notes of encouragement; thanks for your prayers. In Him.

Wednesday, December 31, 2008 7:19 a.m.
Dear friends,

Why ponder the future to foresee;
And jade your brain to vain perplexity?
Cast off your care, leave "God's" plans to Him—
He formed them all without consulting you.
When it is dark enough, you can see the stars.

Two quotes I came across last evening as I began to read *Three Cups of Tea* by Greg Mortenson and David Oliver Relin. I'm not sure where he stands on the theological line, but after changing one word in the third line, they sure meant a lot to me.

As I head over to my PET scan, I pray that I can leave God's plan to Him and see the stars as I look through the darkness.

Thanks for praying.

Wednesday, December 31, 2008 3:14 p.m.
A quick update on mom. She just met with the doctor and the PET scan didn't show anything new so that was the best news that we could have hoped for! She will update more later. Thank you so much for all of your prayers. Mindy

2009

Saturday, January 3, 2009 9:57 p.m.

Dear faithful friends,

I've thought so much about what I would say on my next Caring-Bridge entry that I was surprised when I looked back and saw that the last entry was the one Mindy wrote right after my scan. Somehow I fabricated many stories, but none of them made it to the site.

So many thoughts, so many feelings! So much to comprehend. So much to think about and yet . . . what do I say?

Here's the basics in short form, at least as short as I can say it.

I left you with my anticipated dismissal date from the hospital. The dismissal actually happened on Wednesday morning. I had an early morning visit with Dr. Krie, a quick radiation treatment, my dismissal, and then a PET scan, all by 9:30. (Actually my PET scan began at 9:30.) By noon I felt as if I had already accomplished a lot. I'm thankful that my sister-in-law Shar could pick me up from the hospital and run me over to the scanning building. It is a distance from the hospital so it saved us getting a taxi or having Jerry come up early.

Toward mid-afternoon, my brother-in-law Vern took me to the Cancer Institute where Jerry met me for my visit with Dr. Krie. Jerry and I were nervous. We had read the symptoms so wrong on Friday night that we were scared of what we might find out this time. I wanted badly to believe that my body was free from the cancer the chemo could control. We hardly knew how to react when Dr. Krie told us that she saw no cancer on the PET scan. Nothing! Not a spot! Do you cry? Do you laugh? My heart could only say, "Thank you, Lord!"

Now what's next? Dr. Krie said my case is completely different from any case she has worked with before. In her experience with metastasized breast cancer, the cancer shows up in the protected areas of chemo (the brain and spinal cord) after it has shown up in other parts of the body (lungs, liver, bones). That didn't happen with me. As I understood Dr. Krie to say, she has never seen this before. She has never had a patient with cancer in the protected areas before the unprotected areas. Basically what we will do now is wait. My next MRI is scheduled for March and from there we will make decisions about the next move. If the MRI shows no new growth, we will possibly do nothing. If there is cancerous growth in some area, then we will have to check out other options. Of course, we are hoping and praying for no new growth. We are going to trust that God will keep me "clean" and allow me to continue doing the things He has made me to do. But that is in His hands.

I continue to be amazed at how God has led me through this path. He has comforted me; He has walked with me; He has given me all that I need.

I thank Him every day for all my family, friends, colleagues, students, and those whom I don't even know who have been praying for me and encouraging me in an unbelievable way. Last week Jerry stopped at an old gentleman's place, a widower who lives near Sanborn. The man doesn't get out by himself and relies on others to help him. Jerry stopped to give him a cheery "hello" and deliver some water. The kindly gentleman asked how I was and told Jerry that he prayed for me every day. Every day! What a shock! Every day is like that—people whom I don't even know tell me in some way that they are praying for me. What prayer warriors! Would I do this for others? I'm not sure, but I'd like to think so.

I am very grateful for all of you who continue to remember me in prayer. I must say I do love the personal, encouraging notes or the face-to-face encouragement, but the prayers, the ones God puts on the hearts of His people, are just amazing. How His Spirit must work! In November, my aunt Nancy wrote me a personal note that said, "And as an additional bonus, He gives us brothers and sisters to pray and carry us through—some who we've never met." Just as Romans 8:26-27 says, "In the same way, the Spirit helps us in our weakness. We do not know what we ought to pray for, but the Spirit himself intercedes for us with groans that words cannot express. And he who searches our hearts knows the mind of the Spirit, because the Spirit intercedes for the saints in accordance with God's will."

I thank God and I thank you. In Him.

Tuesday, January 6, 2009 12:57 a.m.

Dear friends,

I am not my own!

That is what my minister said in the introduction to his sermon on Sunday morning. Of course I've heard this statement before—it's part of the creeds our church adheres to. But it struck me differently as I heard it Sunday morning. I'm really not my own! Yes, that concerns what happens here on earth, and more importantly how that affects the end of my life, but somehow it had a different meaning for me this time.

Instead of looking at this statement for the future, I started to look at it as the present. God made me in a special way. He gave me certain strengths and certain weaknesses. All of these are my responsibility. How do I handle them? How do I respond to them? What can I change? What can I not change?

Life is different now. I've learned much about dependence that I don't believe I've understood before. I've always felt pretty self-sufficient but now I realize that my accomplishments and my non-accomplishments are not my own. It is not necessarily because of me, but of whom God has made me to be. He wants me to accomplish things, things I'm probably not even aware of. This probably sounds confusing; it is to me, but it is something I am struggling with right now.

If I belong to God, completely and wholly, then what does He want me to do?

Is this the reason for another setback? I don't know, but my comfort is that I belong, both body and soul, to my faithful and loving Savior Jesus Christ. He watches over me so that not a hair can fall from my head (which isn't many right now) without the will of my Father in heaven. Because I belong to Him, I am assured of eternal life, and that is what makes me willing and ready to live for Him while I serve Him on this earth. I'm looking forward to teaching in another week. That is what I believe God is asking me to do right now—stay faithful as I try to inspire new promising young teachers to serve God in this world.

Today I had my sixth treatment. As before, it went without much ado. My right foot seems to be getting a bit more feeling back and my left foot has only a tinge of numbness. I'm thankful that the numbness has subsided a great deal. I'm still on a pain patch and a few other meds. We'll see when I can cut down on those.

I am not my own. I guess none of us are. But we belong—to our faithful, loving Savior Jesus Christ. Belong.

Thursday, January 8, 2009 10:52 p.m.

Dear friends,

As I lay on my back and listened for the laser to beam my body, all I could think of was "Git um. Git um. Git um." I could imagine myself holding the paddles of the Wii game with my grandsons. Miles is the best. He's always saying, "Ba Ma, come and play with me." Then we pick up the paddles and we try to get to another level by grabbing the stars and the coins, hoping to make ourselves bigger and better. That's what I was shouting in my head, "git um," as I lay as quietly as I could, hoping those beams would hit every spot that needed a shot of radiation.

My radiation ended today. No more rays for now, and we are praying that it stays that way for a long time. When I met with Dr. Schneekloof (oncologist/radiologist), she assured me that 80 percent of people are healed by this treatment. We are praying that I am one of those 80 percent.

Back to my thoughts—Life can be confusing. I still keep coming back to the "who am I" and "I am not my own" questions. If I am not my own, then whose am I? Do I play the gift of life as I play the Wii game? Do I just want to get bigger and better? Is that what I am living for? Am I living for success? As I read through Greg Mortenson's book *Three Cups of Tea*, I once again question my existence. I don't want to live my life as he did—sleeping in the backseat of his old car, La Bambe, tromping on out-of-this-world foot paths, fighting off smugglers, but I do want to contribute to the shalom that God has called each of us to be a part of in His world. Greg did that by building schools in far off places where no one else would go. But how can I do that best? I guess I just have to keep searching and believing that God will lead me in the direction He has planned for me. I want that to be teaching, interacting with my family and friends, touching others' lives through mission work, but we'll see what He wants.

By my last treatment (today) I was hoping to feel more relief from the numbness in my right side, and even though I believe there is some relief, it surely hasn't disappeared. I limp significantly due to weakness on my right side, but it does seem to be subsiding. I always associated limping with muscle or bone involvement but I'm now starting to realize that nerves can have as much to do with it. (Going up steps is not a pretty sight.) I've stopped taking pain pills although I still wear a pain patch. I know from my last experience with radiation on my brain that it did take a bit of time for the symptoms to disappear so I hope this is the case here too. The radiation will continue to work for a few more weeks and then after that I can still assume healing can take place.

Romans 14:8 reminds us that, "If we live, we live to the Lord; and if we die, we die to the Lord. So, whether we live or die, we belong to the Lord."

Thanks again for your faithfulness in encouraging me.

Shalom.

Monday, January 12, 2009 12:28 a.m.

Dear friends,

Sunday morning we had one of my favorite visiting ministers. He's an elderly gentleman who preaches in churches when they need him. At one time he told me he never envisioned himself traveling around to churches after he retired. But he has been one of the biggest blessings in my life (and my family's too). When our kids were in high school and we were without a pastor, the kids decided we really shouldn't look for a minister and just hire Rev. Engbers instead. Well that didn't happen but we still get the blessing of having him occasionally.

Since the morning service was preparatory for communion next Sunday, Rev. Engbers chose a passage that helped us think about how to prepare for this sacrament. The message was based on the first verses of John 13, the passage about being a servant and being willing to wash one another's feet. He stressed that the passage was not about salvation but about how to live right. How we should live as Christ taught and modeled.

My first experience with feet-washing came when we (Michael, Megan, my mom and I) treated ourselves (after being in the bush country of Nigeria for about a week) to a stay in one of the nicest hotels in Abuja. We entered our hotel room at the Hilton and one of the first things we saw in our bathroom was a small basin quite close to the floor. I thought, "My, that's a funny place for a urinal." I didn't know what the funny-looking porcelain basin was. We laughed at ourselves when we discovered what it really was—a foot-washing basin. Why did they have those basins in Abjua and not in the U.S.? Probably because of the dirt, dust, and the heat. There isn't much cement and the dirt is very dusty. Many people in that part of the world wear sandals to keep their feet cool, but to be presentable and clean (which is very important to them) you have to wash your feet. Just as Jesus said to Peter, you don't have to wash your whole body if you've had a bath, but you need only to wash your feet. Peter was confused with Jesus' actions. He didn't understand what Jesus meant—that to be a leader, one must be a servant. Do we? What does that look like to us? How does that transfer into being an employer, an employee, a teacher, a volunteer, a stay-at-home mom? How do we work in God's world as we serve Him by building shalom in His world, serve others and take care of ourselves? That's one of my focuses this week—to be a servant as I lead my students into a better understanding of what it means to be a Christ-filled student.

It was a wonderful weekend. We celebrated Miles' third birthday on

Saturday night. What fun to see a three-year-old open presents and show his appreciation for his gifts. His hugs and kisses were precious. During the party I reflected on the difference between the last party and this one and it was difficult not to wish for my "old" self and to feel "normal" but I keep hoping that feeling will return soon. Over the past few days I believe more feeling is returning to my right leg (my left leg is feeling pretty normal). It is still very numb but there seems to be more strength. I hope this will continue during the next few weeks. I've cut down on some medication and hope tomorrow I can get the go-ahead to cut back on one more.

Thanks again for all your encouragement. Having help with serving cookies in church, receiving notes, words of encouragement, and guest book entries, and most of all, knowing that the prayers of all my prayer warriors are being raised up for me has been an inspiration. As I begin teaching this week, I hope you will join me in prayer that I will be able to do the work of a servant who is trying to bring shalom to this world.

Have a good week.

Monday, January 12, 2009 10:10 p.m.

Dear friends,

Tomorrow is my first day back in class. Usually I wouldn't think of it as a big deal, but after the health issues of the last few weeks, I'm a bit nervous. First of all, the weather has me a little concerned; I hope the roads will be clear. Next I have to worry about getting everything I took home to study, back to my office. I'm not sure I can get it all up the stairs to my office by myself. I'm going to have to be patient and wait for some help—not an easy task for me. I'll pack what I think I need in two bags, one with my computer and the other with books, trying to arrange the weight so it is fairly even. I might have to use the little grips that Kay De Boom bought me for my shoes to help me maneuver the sidewalks. We'll see how this all goes. My strength has increased again today so I hope that will help as I make my way to my office.

Relying on others has never been a strength of mine. I am self-sufficient and I like it that way. Maybe another lesson for me, huh? As I begin my new semester, please pray with me that I can be patient for others to help me, that I can be gracious to those I wait for, and that I can show Christ's love through all of this. Ephesians 4:2 says, "Be completely humble and gentle; be patient, bearing with one another in love." Others are watching. What are they seeing? In Him.

Tuesday, January 13, 2009 10:09 p.m.

Dear friends,

My friend Carolyn Bootsma sent this in the mail today: "Mister Rogers was right after all: There is only one you." It sounds a little egotistical doesn't it? But it isn't. Mr. Rogers wasn't referring to boosting your self-esteem but rather to seeing yourself as unique so you can better serve others by being confident in the God-given role He has planned for our lives.

I Corinthians 12:18 (NLT) says, "God made our bodies with many parts and he has put each part just where he wants it." Just as it is with the human body, so it is with the Body of Christ—we are all a corporate collection of all who believe. Each of us has our own job within God's kingdom. For some of us it is to teach, for some, to be stay-at-home moms, for some businessmen and women, for some, care-takers in care settings. I'm not sure what your job is, but God has appointed you to do the job you have. Sometimes that changes, sometimes not. But wherever He has put you, that is where you are to be faithful. Sometimes we may not feel that we are where we want to be, but it is important to remember that there are no accidents. Whatever we are doing, whatever we are experiencing, we are being shaped to be qualified servants of God's kingdom.

Hurray! I made my first day back at Dordt! It was great to be surrounded by friends, colleagues, and students. My day started out experiencing and accepting help. John Visser was my angel of mercy today. He e-mailed me last night that he would meet me at my building this morning so he could carry my bags into my office. I was very grateful for the help. John's real job may be to teach, but he also used his gifts today to help me. I'm thankful for him and others who serve, for those who help those of us who need help. Another lesson for me—accepting help. I have to say, Jerry has been my other angel of mercy. He's been willing to do the dishes, carry the wash up from the laundry room, pack up my car, and many other things. I came home to find food in the fridge and cards on my table. What a blessing to have those who serve!

Just a thought—are you living for a reason? Are you using your unique gifts to benefit others? In what specific way are you touching others?

There is really no one else like you . . . and that's for a reason. In Him.

Saturday, January 17, 2009 12:53 a.m.

Dear friends,

Slowly, ever so slowly, it seems that some of the side effects of the tumors pressing on the lumbar section of my spine are disappearing. I hope that means the radiation is working. The numbness in my lower back is almost gone. The numbness in my feet is subsiding and my balance and the strength in my legs seem to be improving. Colleagues told me today that they could see great improvement in my walking.

I never assumed it would be like this. I experienced walking difficulties before, when I had my hip replaced, but that was different. There was a real physical problem when I had hip replacement but this time the problem is neurological. The tumors that are pressing on the nerve fibers are causing the numbness and weakness. For some reason this is more difficult for me to accept. Since there is no broken bone, no muscle dysfunction, it doesn't seem as if I should be gimping around, but I am. I'm eager for the day when I don't have to grab the hand-rails to drag myself up the stairs or ride the elevator to get to the second floor. I hope that will come soon. I know all these things help grow character, so as I patiently wait for healing, I'm also going to keep working at that character building.

Matthew 6's bottom line is that we don't have to worry about tomorrow because today has enough troubles of its own. I'm quite aware of that right now. Jesus says that life is often difficult and there is plenty of troubling stuff to consume us. Scott Hozee, in his article "Troubles of the Day," from the winter *Forum*, 2006, says, "Jesus admits that even for the most faithful believer, each day has enough bad stuff as it is, that even the most prayerful person will still lead a life full of difficult realities." Those are the kinds of things that draw us to God, to relying on Him for the things that we need. But as I wait day to day, I also believe I need to be patient as I look ahead. Each day doesn't necessarily bring change but I have seen changes in a week's time and I'm thankful for that. I'm continuing to pray that the healing will continue and that I will have patience to wait for it.

Thanks to all my "angels" this week. Elaine followed me into the parking lot on Wednesday and helped me carry my things upstairs. Kay De Boom and Doug Bonestroo carried my things to my car this afternoon, and there have been others. Thanks for all your help! It's been heart-warming. In Him.

Sunday, January 18, 2009 11:54 p.m.

Dear friends,

Step by step. Little by little. That seems to be the progress I am making. The steps are slow but the progress seems to be in the right direction.

Quite a few years ago, Michael W. Smith produced the song "*Step*

by Step." It was a favorite song of my fourth and fifth grade students at
Sheldon Christian School. The lyrics go like this:

Oh God, You are my God
And I will ever praise You
I will seek You in the morning
And I will learn to walk in Your ways
And step by step You'll lead me
And I will follow You all of my days

I never particularly liked that song, but we sang it often because the
students liked it. I don't think it was the lyrics; possibly it was the tune or
maybe the beat; I don't know. But as I look at those lyrics now, I can see
how important they are in my life. Each step of my life, I am, or at least I
should be, drawn closer to God as He leads me on the journey of my life.

That's what it is, I guess. Step by step God is leading me and I need
to follow—obediently, submissively, but also eagerly and passionately. I
know the song is talking about spiritual steps but as I make these small
physical steps, I can see God working in me there too. At the end of the
week I could reach up on my tippy toes and manipulate the force on the
shower head. Yes, I am "doing" stairs better. Yes, I'm walking stronger.
Yes, all these physical accomplishments show me how God continues to
walk by my side, step by step. I'm thankful for His blessings.

I hope you are experiencing God's leading and guiding step by step
in your life too.

Exodus 15:13 says, "In your unfailing love you will lead the people you have redeemed." That's step by step! Thanks for your continued
prayers and support. Have a good week.

Thursday, January 22, 2009 11:58 p.m.
Dear friends,

Toes . . . tippy toes. I didn't know they had so much importance.
They don't look that powerful. They are just little appendages on the end
of our feet, right? Not really! They have an important job, just as important as other parts of our body. In the past I didn't take notice of what
they did. But I've discovered they are powerful. Just try not having the
ability to reach up with your toes. I'm noticing this as the use of my toes
is coming back. I can now reach up on my toes and shut off the water on
our shower. I have better balance. I can climb steps better, not perfectly
yet, but better. But I've also come to notice something else—I can't keep
my right shoe on my foot. It keeps "slopping" off. I believe my toes have

something to do with that too. I didn't think my shoes were too big when I bought them before this whole new cancer thing cropped up, but I'm beginning to believe that my toes are instrumental in keeping shoes on. Isn't it amazing, the power of your little toes!

God has truly made us unique. He gave each of our body parts a special job to do, even our toes. Psalm 139 says each of us is "fearfully and wonderfully made" by God for service in His kingdom. I'm thankful that God has made me unique; yes, I guess even unique enough that I have the kind of cancer that Dr. Krie has not seen before. I haven't figured this one out yet, but some day it may come clear. We are continuing to pray that the radiation has/is working to shrink the tumors. Today marks two weeks since my last radiation treatment. So now we will have to see what happens. I still have some numbness but it is decreasing somewhat. I'm now struggling with fatigue but I hope that will subside soon too. Please continue to pray with us that the tumors have shrunk, that the cancer can remain at bay, and that energy will return.

Thanks for your cards, words of encouragement, help with dragging my "stuff" to my office and car, for food and most of all, your prayers. We are thankful for all you do. In Him.

Sunday, January 25, 2009 11:33 p.m.
Dear friends,

What a day. I called it my DDD; no Dianne, that doesn't stand for Dordt Discovery Days. Definitely a Delightful Day is what I was thinking of. That was yesterday. Marcia, my twin sister, took me shopping; yes, it is something I love to do but haven't done much of lately. Because my feet are really sore right now, she was even willing to push me around in a wheelchair. I cut down on a pain killer and I'm wondering if that is the reason for my sore feet. My balance and strength have really increased but so has the pain. So we'll have to see how to deal with that.

It was great to get out. I ran into a cousin, a former student, and even a woman who recognized me from my CaringBridge site. It felt good to experience somewhat normal activity once again. I went out for dinner with my sister's family and even took time to stop by my parents and roll up my mom's hair. Yes, she still uses rollers to curl her hair. (Jerry and Josh spent the day at the winter games at Okoboji.) It seems as if my energy is coming back and I'm not suffering as much from fatigue. I'm thankful for that.

As I was leaving Inwood, I noticed a sign by one the churches: "If God is your co-pilot, move over." How simple and yet how profound. I like to think I'm allowing God to be my pilot, but I know that far too often, I try to take the pilot seat. It was a healthy reminder for me to continue to put my reliance on God and let Him lead. As I thought about this, the words of an old familiar hymn came to mind and it seemed to fit well. Here are the words:

Jesus, Savior, pilot me
Over life's tempestuous sea;
Unknown waves before me roll,
Hiding rocks and treacherous shoal.
Chart and compass come from Thee:
Jesus, Savior, pilot me.

"Over life's tempestuous sea . . . .Chart and compass come from Thee: Jesus, Savior, pilot me."

During the past two years, my life has had a few tempestuous "seas." Sometimes when I think about what has happened over the past years, I can hardly believe that all of this really happened to me. Diagnosis of cancer, mastectomy, chemo treatments, infusions, and then oral medication, PET scans, brain tumors, surgery, radiation, MRIs, lumbar tumors, more radiation. All in two years. And now once again waiting; waiting to see the effects of the radiation. "Unknown waves before me roll." I'm sometimes scared about the future. Nothing seems to follow the normal path for me. My PET scans have been fantastic, but my protected areas have been affected. How can this be? I don't know, but I do know that God has a "chart and a compass" for me. He is my pilot and I will continue to trust in Him. I hope you will too. In Him.

Tuesday, January 27, 2009 11:14 p.m.

Big C, little c, what begins with C? Is it a cheer; is it a rap; is it a question?

When Marcia and I were little, we used to love to play "pretend." We would sit on the upstairs steps and play pretend church. Or we would play pretend beauty shop. (Once we even got in the car and pretended to drive to the pretend beauty shop where we proceeded to cut off the hair of one of our lovely dolls—not pretend. She was forever bald, just like me.) Sometimes we would pretend to cheerlead. Maybe that's what the Big C, little c reminded me of, cheering.

Or maybe not. As I came across it today in one of my devotionals, I was reminded of what it should stand for. Big C, little c. I know that sometimes I concentrate too much on the Big C standing for cancer. I feel and see what it has done to me, how it has altered my life, how it has made me change many of the things I've always been able to do or desire to do. But today as I read a devotional from one of my favorite books, I was reminded that I have to think of the Big C as Christ and the little c as cancer. The words I read were a reminder of where the fullest healing power lies—in our Lord Jesus Christ. I pray that I will deepen my desire to live for Him as I cope with this cancer diagnosis and all its realities. It is difficult to live with the unknowns and face things of which I am not in control. Things like headaches, muscle pain, numbness, all the little aches and pains; it's scary. But what a blessing to know that Christ is walking with me each step of the way, with each breath that I breathe, with each blink that I blink. Nothing happens without Him knowing. I pray that I can continue to focus on Christ as my big C and let Him crush the little c. And through all this, I hope I glorify God.

"When I am afraid, I will trust in you. In God, whose word I praise, in God I trust; I will not be afraid" (Psalm 56:3-4).

Thanks again for all your support. Today we received more food and cards. We had delicious soup from Kay and a card all the way from our friend Hazel in Florida. What a blessing to feel and receive the communion of the saints! In Him.

February 1, 2009 2:15 p.m.

Hello dear friends,

I have to tell you about my experience with a "Garden of Delight" last night: well, really this weekend. On Friday night my grand-nephew wrestled in town so we had the delight of watching him win his two matches, and then he and some of my family came for supper. We had a delightful time eating, conversing, and laughing together. We haven't had guests over much during the past few months so it was fun to entertain once again. (Of course, they brought most of the food which made it easy for me.) Then on Saturday evening, after much anticipation, we were taken out by some of our best friends. Nate Breen had told us weeks ago to reserve January 31. We weren't sure what that was going to entail; we were curious and excited to see what he had planned. At 5:30 a vehicle pulled up to pick us up. In it were our friends Nate and Cath, Nate and MaryBeth, and John and Amy. We got in the vehicle and were taken to dinner at the Blue Mountain in Orange City. The dinner was great but the conversation and company were even greater. Since August when I was diagnosed with my brain tumors and then later with my lumbar tumors, we haven't socialized much, so it was wonderful to sit and chat with friends in a wonderful environment. (We had the zebra room all to ourselves.) We didn't feel any need to hurry, so our dinner lasted about four hours. In fact, the guys had to come up twice to tell us it was time to leave because we just couldn't quit talking. We finally got in the vehicle and continued talking until we reached Sanborn. What a delightful night!

God blesses us in many ways. Friends are one of them. Yes, we enjoyed a great night out with friends last night, but we have been blessed by many people. Yesterday we received an invitation to come visit some friends in Arizona. We have received wonderful cards from people all over the country. Some are from people with whom we have established friendships, others we know only by name and still others are those who have heard about my cancer and in Christian love have reached out to us. It is amazing how many people remind us that they are praying not only for me, but our whole family. Friends are an important part of all of our lives. Proverbs 17:17 says, "A friend loves at all times." The commentary that described this verse says there is vast difference between knowing someone and being a true friend. I Corinthians 13:7 adds that a friend " . . . always protects, always trusts, always hopes, always perseveres." This verse indicates that even though it goes against our sinful nature, God can indeed help us set aside our own desires so that we can show our love without expecting anything in return.

It was the same message we heard this morning in church. We looked at Heidelberg Catechism, Lord's Day 3, which says—by God's grace we are born again, He can turn our actions into good. The interpretation of the verse says that the more we are like Christ, the more we can show love to others. Sometimes we are like fair-weather friends; when the going gets tough, we bow out. We leave when folks run into hardships or we don't think we are getting what we should out of a relationship. In thinking of my friendships, I know that I have sometimes been that kind of friend. But I must say the benefits we have received from friends, both close friends and acquaintances, both near and far, have been unbelievable. You have blessed us in many ways. I hope I can always be a friend that protects, trusts, hopes, and perseveres. How about you?

As far as my health, each day I do get stronger. That may sound silly to you—how can I keep getting stronger? But I do. I still struggle with stair steps, but I'm getting better. I don't need to use the arm rails as much. I'm walking faster—ask my colleagues. My toes are stronger; my leg muscles can push more.

Thanks for all your support. We appreciate all the big and little things you have done for us.

I hope you have a great week! I'm looking forward to some great teaching moments and being a good friend. In Him.

Sunday, February 8, 2009 11:31 p.m.

Dear friends,

Wanna skip? Wanna jog? Wanna run? Well, maybe not with me, but I'm getting close to being able to do some of the things I used to be able to do. I'm not ready to run a race but I'm becoming stronger in my walking and in the use of my legs. I continue to be amazed at what my legs, feet, and toe muscles do. I've had great help again this week. Doug shows up every morning to carry my things to the office; Ed carried my things down this week; I met Leah in the hallway and she volunteered to help me, and Kay always asks if she can help. I work with a wonderful bunch of people.

As I said, I'm not ready to run a race right now, at least not to win one. But I am ready to run the race that God has put before me. Sometimes I feel overwhelmed with all that has come my way. Sometimes I still question all that I'm going through. Tonight the word race caught my attention so I began looking up verses that connected with the word race. At first I looked up some of the verses where Paul talked about running the race, but then I turned to Ecclesiastes. When I read the introduction I discovered that the purpose of the book was to spare future generations from bitterness when they learned that life is meaningless apart from God.

The author told the story about a little boy who received an Easter bunny. I imagine it was one of those cute little bunnies that we see on the shelves at Easter. The ones we buy and lay in a basket filled with green grass. The little boy takes a bite, anticipating a nice chunk of chocolate and finds instead something hollow, empty. Something that just falls apart when bitten into. My commentary said, "Empty, futile, hollow, nothing . . . the words ring of disappointment and disillusionment. Yet this is the life-experience of many. Grasping the sweet things—possessions, experience, power, and pleasure—they find nothing inside. Life is empty, meaningless, and they despair." Ecclesiastes has a negative tone, but it isn't meant to discourage but to lead people to seek true happiness in God. When I read Ecclesiastes 9:11, I wondered how to interpret it. It says, "The race is not to the swift or the battle to the strong, nor does food come to the wise or wealth to the brilliant or favor to the learned; but time and chance happen to them all." It goes on to say in verse 12:

"Moreover, no man knows when his hour will come: As fish are caught in a cruel net, or birds are taken in a snare, so men are trapped by evil times that fall unexpectedly upon them." Again, the commentary reminded me that the swift don't always win the race. You remember seeing sure winners trip just before the finish line. I remember having one of the fastest times going into a state race when I was a senior in high school only to find that they changed some rules which we weren't informed of and I ended up disqualifying my team. What a devastating feeling! We all know brilliant people whose intelligence hasn't rewarded them with wealth or honor. Life isn't always fair. But the point Solomon is trying to make here is that because life isn't fair, we need to look to God for our hope. None of us knows how long our life will be. Someone reminded me that even though they are healthy now, their life could end before mine. None of us knows the number of our days. That's why God tells us to use each day wisely and proclaim His glory each and every day. I wonder what that will look like in my life this week. How about yours? Have a good week.

P.S. I'm going down on steroids this week, so please pray that I can stay strong and teach well.

Monday, March 9, 2009 7:06 p.m.

I want to update and let everyone who hasn't heard know that mom is in the hospital. They found a spot on the MRI that Dr. Krie was concerned with. Mom is scheduled to have surgery tomorrow at 3:00 to put in a reservoir to receive chemo for the spot. This reservoir will be under the skin on her head. They then will use this device to put the chemo in to get it directly into her system. I'm sure she will update later, but I thought I'd let you all know what we know as of now. Thank you for all of your thoughts and prayers. Mindy

Thursday, March 12, 2009 2:15 p.m.

Finally, an update. I know many have been curious how mom is doing. The last week has been, well, we're still trying to make sense of it.

Saturday mom went to the ER in Sioux Falls with a lot of pain and difficulty swallowing and even talking. Anyone who knows Cella knows difficulty talking means something is wrong! After a CT scan and MRI, they discovered cancer in the lining of the brain (best way I can think to describe it), a spot deep in her brain, and a tiny spot in her lung. Dr. Krie said she is not worried about the lung at this point. It could grow and grow and not affect mom for quite some time. Dealing with the other spot and the fluid is a bit trickier. Dr. Krie stressed that she is focusing on the quality of mom's life at this point, not quantity. Our best option to deal with this started Tuesday with mom's surgery. An ommaya reservoir was implanted in the brain to administer the chemotherapy. Because of the protective barrier surrounding the brain, it makes administering chemo to these desired sites more complicated. The ommaya reservoir is a plastic, dome-shaped device implanted under the skin at the top of the head, with a catheter (thin tubing) attached to the underside used to deliver chemotherapy to the desired spots. (If you want more information on the ommaya reservoir, you can read a bit more here: http://www.answers.com/topic/ommaya-reservoir.)

The surgery was quite minor compared to her last surgery. The incision is small and we couldn't believe how good it looked Tuesday night already! She is quite sleepy and they are working on figuring out the proper balance for her pain meds. Monday she was in quite a bit of pain. Tuesday she was a bit over-medicated. Wednesday she was able to swallow better and her voice was stronger when she talked. They are hoping to administer the first dose of chemo today sometime. They will observe how she reacts to the treatment and will then determine if she can go home or if she'll stay through the next treatment.

So what does the future hold? We have no idea. We do know this diagnosis is different than the others. We are hoping the chemo will relieve some of her current symptoms: the difficulty of swallowing and talking and the pain that brought her into the ER. We are still praying for a miracle cure. We know God can do anything. I am confident that no matter how He answers our prayers, He will give us the peace that passes understanding as we walk through this next valley in mom's journey. As a family, we are focusing on making the best decisions we can make, leaving the results of the chemo in God's hands and doing our part of living faithfully with however much time we have left. No matter if we have a month or year or five years, we have stories to laugh through, fun to be had, and memories to make. We have had many tears as we've imagined the future and shared our fears. But we've had equal amounts of laughter. The hospital can make an already loopy family even loopier!

Mom has been very tired and her voice is still gaining in strength. We need to be careful of the germs she is exposed to and her current energy level. It's hard to turn away visitors because she thrives on the encouragement and love she gets in many different ways! If you are wondering about a visit, it is best to call dad on his phone before planning a trip. Her voice is getting stronger but it also might be best if you call dad's phone to see if she is strong enough to talk on the phone. If you do visit or call, it is best for mom to make your hellos to her brief. She started out with a pretty strong voice this morning but currently can only whisper. There is a waiting room where dad often goes to talk longer with visitors after they say hello to mom. Other ways you could show her love or support during this time? She loves getting cards and notes on her CaringBridge site. I think she's kept every card she's received since her initial breast cancer diagnosis. As noted above, we aren't sure exactly how long she'll still be in the hospital. If she responds well to the chemo today, she could go home as early as this evening or Friday morning. If she does not, she could be staying through the weekend.

We will be sure to update with her status of going home or staying in the hospital longer as they monitor her tolerance of the chemotherapy treatment so you know where to show and send your love. We'll be sure to post an address once we know how long she'll be in the hospital. Please note that no flowers are allowed on her wing. Big bummer . . . Cella loves flowers!

We thank you all for your concerns, thoughtfulness, and prayers. We continue to experience the church at work in very humbling ways. Megan

Thursday, March 12, 2009 11:54 p.m.

Chemotherapy went very well today. She did not experience any headaches or other symptoms. A huge blessing.

Despite the good chemotherapy run, mom's health continues to decline. Her voice got weaker throughout the day. Mustering out a whisper is quite a feat. She has coughed a lot throughout the day, breathing has become difficult as well, and she is restless. Dr. Krie stopped in this evening and said she was worried, something she's never said before. She said that if the chemo does not start to reverse some of these difficulties, she's worried she's started the active phase of dying. Mom fades in and out of conversation. She often makes sense but sometimes appears confused and wants reassurance where she is.

Mindy and Sou, Josh, and Mike all joined my dad and me for the evening. Mom keeps saying she doesn't want to die but she is tired of feeling this way. She asks, "Does Dr. Krie think I'm dying?" Tells us, "I don't want to die. I just don't want to die." It's hard to know how to respond.

We are praying fervently for a lack of pain for mom right now and for wisdom for us in knowing how to reassure and answer the questions she asks us, in and out of her sleep. One thing we know for sure, she's very adamant she does not want funeral food when she does die. It's been a meaningful evening. We keep asking for God's grace as we cherish every moment we get together.

We are not sure how long mom will be at the hospital. If you do come to visit, visits are limited to one to five minutes. Dad really appreciates the support and company but mom does not have the energy to talk or listen to conversation at this point.

We know God is doing the most loving thing concerning us during these hours. Megan

Friday, March 13, 2009 4:42 p.m.

Visitor update:

Mom has not been up to visitors today. She tires out very quickly. Dad appreciates visitors very much. If you would like to visit the hospital this evening or throughout the weekend, you can find dad or another family member in the waiting area/lounge in her wing. (You may have to call dad if you need directions or specifics . . . unfortunately, I got my mom's sense of direction.) Depending on how mom is feeling, visitors may be allowed to say hi for a minute or two. Much more than that is very difficult for her to tolerate. We appreciate knowing how much everyone cares for and loves mom.

Today's update:

Mom had a rough night last night. She talked about death often and had a lot of anxiety. Today, her voice continues to be a whisper at its strongest. She has not eaten in a few days and is sleeping a lot. She will sometimes be confused but she still cracks jokes and uses the biggest words she can when she needs to get messages out. She said it was "very cordial of Erik to call" when someone from Dordt called and told me that when I get to heaven, it will be the most organized place ever . . . a complete nightmare. We've been amazed how much she can communicate just through her eyes! She can clearly express "Don't be stupid" to "Wow that was too much" to "I just hate this."

Mom knows what a beautiful place heaven is, totally void of pain and suffering, but death is still scary. She's a fighter. She always has been and always will be to her very last breath. Even through her whispers and struggles for breath, she is fighting. The doctors have commented that they think she's been fighting a lot longer than any of us were aware of. Does that surprise us one bit? We've wondered with mom how amazing it will be for her to hear the words "Well done my good and faithful servant" when she gets to heaven. For me, it's been a comfort to imagine my mom's entrance into heaven being greeted with those words. She has been a radiant model of faith and service.

We have loved reading stories that people have been sending in. One of mom's fears in dying is not being present in her grandchildren's lives. We have started compiling the stories that are shared so we can have tangible ways to always remember with our kids how faithful their grandma walked, how much fun she had in life, and how many countless lives she has touched. Feel free to share stories you might have of how she has touched your life, a funny memory, or anything else that might help us remember. Remembering is an amazing way to celebrate the life God has created in mom.

Today mom whispered to Barb Hoekstra, "I've had a wonderful life." We think it's been quite extraordinary. Megan

Saturday, March 14, 2009 2:55 p.m.

Cella has always kept everyone on their toes . . . yesterday was no exception.

Thursday night was horrible. Even she thought she was going to die. Friday morning was filled with finding meds to ease pain and anxiety. Mid-morning to early afternoon she was able to sleep a lot. And then, tenacious Cella started to show some spunk. She ate a few bites of mashed potato, visited briefly with her grandkids, and started to ask why she thought she was going to die the night before. Her color looked better. Her voice was a little stronger. It was amazing! We all wondered if it was the chemo starting to work or if it was due to some of the new medications. No matter what the cause of her turn for the better, we know all those prayers going up on her behalf have something to do with it. Our God is amazing!

She had a ton of visitors on Friday afternoon through the evening. She was able briefly to say hello to every visitor and was honored that people were remembering her. She's always surprised that people continue to think of her.

If you plan to visit today, we ask that you first sign her guest book in the lounge/waiting area and talk to a family member to see if she is up for visitors. We want to conserve as much energy as she needs to get healthy. We will post these reminders on her door, but also please keep in mind to wash your hands before going into her room, turn off your cell phones before entering her room, limit your visits from one to three minutes, and remember to talk quietly. It's best to do most of the talking rather than ask mom questions. Right now, we are recommending not to take children into her room.

We'll keep you updated on how this most wonderful wife, mom, grandma, daughter, sister, teacher and friend of all continues to keep us on our toes. Megan

Monday, March 16, 2009 10:21 p.m.

Saturday evening mom was in quite a bit of pain. Sunday was pretty steady with no change.

Today, mom continues to struggle with a weak voice, a lack of muscle strength in her throat to swallow, pain in her back, and phlegm that she works very hard to cough out. The doctors stopped in this morning and noted the chemo that started last week Thursday does not seem to be making a difference. She has continued to decline since she was admitted into the hospital. She received another chemo treatment today to see if another dose will make a difference and at the same time we have decided to move forward with hospice. Mom will be moving to the Dougherty Hospice House in Sioux Falls tomorrow at some point. It was very difficult for mom to make this decision with us. She felt that it was a place for old people and really felt as if she was giving up by accepting hospice. After we as a family took a tour and reported what a truly amazing place this is, mom said "sign me up." We believe this facility will be able to bring more enjoyment and freedom to mom during her last days of life. She can have flowers in her room, has a beautiful and spacious room with a better sleeping option for dad, and can focus on her spiritual and emotional health in addition to maintaining her comfort with all of her current medications.

The move to the Dougherty House is going to take a lot of energy for mom. Just going to the bathroom or changing clothes completely wipes her out. Here are a few ways you can pray for her and us:

- strength for the move from the hospital to this facility
- the ability to enjoy and transition to her new surroundings
- strength and energy for all of us supporting mom—to enjoy every moment we can,
- take care of ourselves
- peace for mom. She continues to have a fear of dying.

We continue to be uplifted and encouraged as you sign her guest book. It's been fun laughing through some of the stories shared in the guest book and in person at the hospital. As I type this, the lounge is filled with laughter reflecting on a vacation we took to New York City when we kids were about middle-school age. We had missed our tour bus but saw a greyhound plowing down the street. In absolute excitement we had found our bus, the entire Vern and Shar Anema family and our family chased down the bus. To our amazement, the bus stopped in the middle of traffic and all ten of us piled in, so proud of our street smarts. The brilliant tourists that we were, the last person on the bus remembered to ask if the bus was indeed going to our destination. You guessed it . . . not all greyhounds were destined to the location we were headed to. It was like on TV . . . we all piled out accompanied by swearing in all kinds of languages with trash flying at us through the air. That only touches the surface of the adventure that vacation provided.

Thanks for your prayers as we continue to love mom in the very best ways we can. Megan

Tuesday, March 17, 2009 10:11 p.m.

We are moved. Mom was tired but did the trip really well. She is settled in her new room and is surrounded with the fresh aroma of FLOWERS. Her face lights up with delight every time a new bouquet is delivered to her room. We love seeing mom light up. Thank you to those of you who sent flowers.

Mom is as impressed with the Dougherty House as we are. Her suite has two adjoining rooms. One room for the patient and one room for a family room/sleeping room. It has been a blessing already to have a little more room as a family. We are planning to use the adjoining room for rest for our immediate family and for those who sit with mom when we need a break. Mom continues to get a lot of company. We cannot guarantee visits to mom if you plan to visit as she sleeps a lot and is still struggling with nausea and pain. But dad absolutely loves the company.

There are several waiting rooms/common rooms in this facility. Mom is in suite 15. You can either check the sign on her door to see where family is planted for the day or talk to someone at the nurses' station located just before her suite. They will be able to advise where you can wait for a family member to meet you. There is a guest book outside the door that we would love to have you sign. Mom is very sensitive to noise, especially when she is sleeping. We want to respect her need for quiet and rest when she needs it.

Within the course of today, Amira and Nico (Cella's grandkids from Nigeria) were able to have some quality time with grandma. They made thumb prints with sculpey clay and had fun decorating grandma's room to make it pretty. Tomorrow Mindy is planning on taking her boys up to have some quality time with grandma when she is awake. The three oldest grandkids especially have many questions and are processing a lot.

We've been praying for wisdom as we meet mom's needs, our children's needs, and the needs of daily life still going on around us. One of the things mom has said repeatedly since she was admitted a little over a week ago is that she wants to enjoy her grandchildren. It's hard because her energy level is low and our kids' energy level is high. Even though the interactions are brief, we want to make them as meaningful as we can. If you have any ideas to share that you've done with children in such a situation, we'd love to hear them.

To the Dougherty House: When coming from Iowa, take 26th Street, turn left at the Bahnson Street stoplight. Turn right onto 52nd Street. About a block down 52nd, you will see an Avera sign for Prince of Peace and Dougherty House. Turn right onto Prince of Peace Place, veering left towards the lodge-looking building.

We'll try posting pictures of mom's new set-up soon. Thanks for your continued prayers . . . for mom and all of us! Megan

Thursday, March 19, 2009 3:01 a.m.

I'm doing this Cella-style tonight . . . I should be totally in bed but can't sleep so I thought I would update since many have said they appreciate knowing her current status.

Mom remained steady today. No improvements but no declines either. She rested very well last night. We all did actually. It was wonderful! Mindy and Sou arrived with their boys in the morning and had really meaningful moments with mom. The boys made fingerprints with sculpey clay, Mindy read books with the kids and grandma, and when her energy level got too low, the boys went outside her window and blew bubbles. She couldn't stop smiling. To be able to watch her grandkids play from the comfort of her bed was a blessing for her today!

Other highlights in mom's day were: More flowers! Seriously, it smells like a garden in her room. The bell! If we are sitting on the couch, it can be difficult telling when mom is awake or sleeping. Since whispering is a chore, she can't let us know with her voice that she is awake. Aunt Marcia (mom's twin sister) brought up a bell from her house so that mom can ring the bell if we are in the room but not aware she has awakened. A new control she is thoroughly enjoying! When the bell was first brought up, mom and dad did a little test to see how far dad could hear it ring. After all test rings were finished, dad went to pull out his bed for the night. He heard a ring only a minute after leaving her room and raced back in, asking what she needed. Mom whispered, "Nothing. It just works really good." Weak? Yes. Feisty still? Definitely!

We continue to be very cautious with visitors. Mom is still very weak and even five minute interactions can send her to sleep for a few hours. We want to remind her loyal friends and family members that we cannot guarantee visits to mom at this time. Dad loves to share stories and appreciates the company very much. Mom keeps reminding us that he's never been much of a sitter. If you come for a visit, you can let the nurses who are stationed right before her room know that you are here so that they can inform us. We prefer to meet all visitors in one of the lounge areas. (There is a dining area, a piano area and one other waiting area I believe.) Once the nurses let us know visitors have arrived, we will find you. We are finding that we kids and my dad are needing a "safe place" to unwind, create special memories with our children, and keep mom's environment quiet and peaceful. Thank you for helping us do this when you visit. It's one of the best ways we can love mom right now. Megan

Friday, March 20, 2009 7:20 a.m.

Mom never liked roller coasters. The older I get, the less of a fan I've become of roller coasters. Our entire family is vouching for our dislike for the current roller coaster we are riding in life.

The peaks are amazing, but the rush to the bottom often leaves us speechless and exhausted. Yesterday was filled with those peaks and rushes. At 5 a.m. Dad called Mindy, who stayed overnight in Sioux Falls. Mom's breathing was shallow and things started to look as they did a week ago on Thursday when mom thought she was going to die. Once Mindy arrived, mom requested she call me (I had gone home to tuck my kids into bed in Sioux Center and was planning to have a day at home to get caught up). By 7:30, Josh, Mindy, and I were all at her bedside. It's tough seeing her in her valleys. Dad got a clipboard so she could write messages down. Her mind is just racing with thoughts, ideas, and to-do lists. She seemed a bit more relaxed once we were all there and she had gotten a few messages out. And she then was able to sleep.

After a few hours of sleep and quiet time, she woke up quite perky. We sang songs together and she asked to listen to music, a first since being hospitalized. In the afternoon we rode the roller coaster to experience a few peaks. In the middle of visiting with someone, she requested a sip of Diet Coke. She said she wanted to chug it but promised to take only a sip of a thickened Diet Coke. (All her liquids are thickened to reduce risks of choking and aspirating.) She then requested a mouse-size nibble of a truffle one of her chemo docs handmade for her. And then she asked for chocolate ice cream with marshmallow on top, Culvers-style. Granted, all of these "bites" were smaller than baby-size, but she was asking. And she was able to swallow it all! We are hoping today we can try a few more foods. She really hasn't eaten since she was admitted to the hospital almost two weeks ago. Whenever someone visits, she asks if they are going shopping and where they are going to eat.

So pray for more success in eating today, grace for the ups and the downs, and the ability for us all to celebrate God's gift of life to the full.

Visitors are still welcome, but with mom's predictable ups and downs, again, we cannot guarantee if anyone will be able to see mom. Megan's kids are coming in the afternoon to make a few more memories with grandma so we will be reserving some energy for that today. Dad is always up to chatting and loves to get out of the facility when we are around for mom. Megan

Sunday, March 22, 2009 1:00 a.m.

Not a lot of changes today. Mom did sleep more but when she was awake, she was pretty alert. She ate a bit of a push-up but nothing more than previous days.

Mom has been sharing some wisdom/life stuff with us the past week. One question we asked went something like this: "What do you like most about your job?" Mom responded in whispers and writing to reveal what a joy it is to have students come back and thank her. She loves knowing that she made a difference in their lives and hearing how they are now living their life. She was stunned to see visitors who drove up from Indiana today. They weren't former students directly from the classroom, but they did go on several serve projects to Cary, Mississippi, with her and no doubt all grew through that experience. Mom was a fan of teaching and impacting but she was also a fan of being a learner herself. She learned much from her students!

We have no way of predicting what kind of day she'll have tomorrow (Sunday) so we cannot guarantee even short visits or peeking your head in to say hello. If you do get to see mom, she wrote yesterday that "yes and no questions are best for someone in my condition."

Mike and my kids took dad out for lunch today. His sister and other Sanborn friends took him out for supper tonight. It's tough to get him away from mom's side but it has been healthy for him to have breaks outside of the facilities where she is staying. He appreciates much all the snacks that are sent, the notes on CaringBridge and in the mail, and those of you who have taken him out. We all cannot say enough thanks for the prayers that continue to carry us. Megan

Sunday, March 22, 2009 11:18 p.m.

Mom slept a little more today. Her facial muscles seem to be getting weaker. She tried to get in the wheelchair to visit the waiting room but only made it through her door before she motioned that she was tired and needed to get back in bed. She continues to fight. Prayers you can lift for mom: peaceful rest, no pain, for a peace that passes understanding as her journey of life on earth comes to a close.

Today we gave out the award to the visitor who has traveled the most miles to see mom. Yesterday, Russ and Mary showed up from Indiana. Today, my cousin Kent, his wife Rachelle, and son Simon showed up from New Mexico! (We'll get you your award later Kent!)

As kids and teenagers, we would sometimes complain about having to share our mom with so many people. So many people have considered her to be like their own mom. Even today at church, a woman commented on how so many people consider mom their best friend, even after just meeting her for a few minutes. She had that effect on people. Yes, sharing our time had some sacrifices, but those sacrifices were met by many more blessings than we would have had sticking to ourselves. Seeing my mom and dad live with an open door to their home and their hearts has greatly impacted all three of us kids. In my own life, I track my own love for people and community to the ways I saw my mom live on a day-to-day basis. Our home was always open. She took seriously the command to "love your neighbor as yourself" and was always reaching out to others. She didn't always feel like going to events or doing the things she did, but she often persevered and was most always blessed by choosing to invest in kingdom-building activities rather than pleasure activities for herself. I'm not saying there is no room for pleasure. We are trying to take time for ourselves during this very journey to make sure we are healthy in every way possible. I do find in America that it is easy to overly invest in ourselves and ignore the groaning needs around us. Often, it doesn't take much time. A word of appreciation here. A thoughtful note there. Sometimes, it is simply looking up and noticing the needs around us. Living a life filled with care for others makes for an incredibly rich life. There is much more I would love to share and ponder on this issue, but fatigue is taking over my brain.

We are all doing well, very thankful for the moments we continue to get with mom, but we are all getting a little tired. Prayers for strength for the journey for our family would be appreciated. Megan

Tuesday, March 24, 2009 2:27 a.m.

It's amazing to get a glimpse into the mind of a child. Amira, Cella's granddaughter, had a program this evening. Mindy and I switched places in the Dougherty House so that I could go home to celebrate Amira's first program at Sioux Center Christian by hitting the bakery after school before we got ready for the big event. We were talking about grandma while we ate our doughnuts. Amira shared her amazement that everyone in her school knew her grandma. "Even the third graders Mom!" She was trying to make sense of how all these people knew her grandma when she exclaimed, "It's like she won the Piston Cup or something!" (The big race on the cartoon movie *Cars*.) I can't wait to continue to share stories with Amira as she gets older so she can more fully understand who her amazing grandma was.

Last week we were called up to Sioux Falls early in the morning when mom wasn't looking so good. I wrote a note to Amira explaining why I was gone and that this might be the day when grandma got to meet Jesus. When I got home later that day, I told Amira how grandma had asked for Diet Coke and ice cream. Instead of excitement for her sudden perkiness, she gave me a deeply dissatisfied look and said, "I thought you said she was going to meet Jesus today!"

Both my sister's and my kids have been asking lots of questions and talking a lot about grandma. But even in their love for grandma, there is a child-like enthusiasm for meeting Jesus that sometimes we lose as adults. It was good for me to hear Amira's excitement for mom to meet Jesus.

Mom slept almost the entire day today. I had about five minutes of awake time with her today and Mindy had five minutes of awake time with her this evening. She is having a more difficult time writing messages and is starting to appear more confused. A bad day? A sign that the end is getting closer? Not sure. We'll just continue to love her to the best of our ability until she does get to be with Jesus. We are all praying for grace for the moments, especially when the last moment comes. Megan

Thursday, March 26, 2009 10:04 a.m.

"It's not fair." It's a common phrase we've heard and battled against in our house. When Amira was three, she knew enough not to say the entire battle-inducing phrase, but would occasionally test the waters with a "It's not f, f, f, f, ..." Nico, another one of Cella's grandchildren, recently caught on to the phrase. I think I've heard Mindy's boys echo the same sentiment as well since we've arrived in Iowa.

Yesterday, I have to admit that the phrase crossed my mind as I watched mom: unable to respond with voice, whisper, or motions. The sound of the "death rattle" was in her lungs as she coughed. Her breath came irregularly. Her eyes were glassy and no longer closed when she slept or indicated if she understood. When she could no longer raise her hand to her head, I thought "this is just not fair." It's not fair that cancer robs life right out from under a person. It's just not fair.

And as these thoughts ran through my mind, I held my mom's hand, I tapped into my mommy-mental-coach, reminding myself that life indeed is not fair. I'm not sure why we are surprised by that. Sometimes it's easy to think that as Christians, we deserve more in life. But we were never promised a fair or easy life. Just because we believe does not mean that blessing after blessing will fall into our lap. Not in the way the world thinks of blessings anyway: wealth, good health, success in all we do, freedom from hardship, etc. Simply believing in Jesus Christ as our Savior does not save us from the pain and hardship that accompany life. I'm sure many of mom's readers have plenty of their own stories of pain and difficulty that attest to the truly rough road many Christians travel. I echo Amira in her shout the other day in utter grief for grandma's approaching death: "I just wish those people didn't eat that apple!" We weren't promised a pain-free life but we were promised New Life. So while we aren't free from experiencing the effects of sin such as pain or sadness or death, we do have free access to the promises offered in the Bible. Mom would be able to quote you verse and chapter where these promises come in the Bible. Right now, I'm drawing blanks and am too tired to search and find proof of some of the promises that come to my mind. I do know that God will never leave us or forsake us. He knows our pain and empathizes with us. He meets our every need and will never allow more than we can handle. He loves us unconditionally. And after we persevere down the road that He calls us, we are greeted with eternal life.

We are clinging to those promises and many more that the Bible gives us that I'm not recalling at this moment. We wish we had a road map right about now, telling us more specifically how to walk down this path. Since we don't, we cling to the instructions and promises given to us throughout the Bible. And we pray that God helps us walk faithfully, honestly, and in a way that brings glory to His name.

One of my kids' favorite Hausa songs goes something like this: Ni zan je de Yesu ko ina. Ban damu da gargada hanya ba. Ni zan je, ni zan je. I must go with Jesus anywhere, no matter the roughness of the road. I must go. I must go. So thankful we have someone like Jesus to walk this road with us. It can be a rough road, but no matter what the state of the road we travel, in the end, we meet a glorious end. Mom is almost there. Megan

Thursday, March 26, 2009 11:31 p.m.

We nominated dad to take over the CaringBridge updates but figured mom's friends might not be able to take his cliff-hanger, to-be-continued style of story telling. We had a good laugh as a family as we discussed and reminisced about dad's infamous story-telling tactics.

Mom is hanging on. She's moving to days and hours. It's hard to know where to be as we wait. We've been starting to plan how we will grieve the loss and celebrate mom's life through visitation and funeral services. We have to decide on many details and arrangements. Megan

Sunday, March 29, 2009 9:35 a.m.

Have you ever experienced a situation or event where you wanted to fast-forward? You knew you could get through, and you knew that God was probably going to teach you something through it. But you wanted to get to the end when it was all over because you had already grown and could move on?

I have this feeling in the airport a lot. Our last few moments after checking in baggage to the dreaded walk through security with final waves and thrown-kisses is torture for me. No matter who it is, our Mt. View Hostel kids, our siblings, or our parents—I tend to want to fast-forward to those last precious moments, past pain and the awkwardness of the good-byes, and move on.

That's a bit how we are feeling right now.

These last few days have been difficult. We are loving mom as much as we can. But it's hard to talk and sing and read scripture when we have no idea how much she is hearing us or how much she is even wanting that interaction. Can you imagine sitting all alone with no-one talking to you because you couldn't respond? Or could you imagine having someone talk your ear off when all you wanted is silence? With those thoughts in mind, we do know that God is probably talking to and comforting mom in ways we cannot even begin to imagine. It's hard to know if we should go home at night or, in case this is "the night," to stay. It's hard not to think about the impending funeral and busy ourselves with plans when mom is still here. It's hard to wait.

And yet we know God doesn't merely have us in a holding pattern. There is a reason mom's heart is still fairly strong even though the rest of her body is struggling and failing. God isn't quite finished yet, with her or with us.

As we walk these last few days, we are trying to be open to the whispers we are hearing from God. We are trying to enjoy our moments of silence with mom, holding her hand and stroking her smooth face.

I was chatting online with a global Child-life Specialist advocate last night and she sent me this poem:

"We do not have the wide-angle, all-encompassing vision of God. Our losses hurt, our pain is real. We are not healed by being told that God's timing is best, that heaven is a better place, that our loved one has been spared suffering. We are healed by being breathed back to life with love that only the breath of God can give" (Joanna Lufer and Kenneth S. Lewis).

It urged me to face the fact that even though we are ready for mom to enter heaven, it's not going to make it easy. These last few days, as hard as it is to see mom like this, will not fully prepare us for her final breath and departure.

My husband Mike is preaching and sharing about our work in Nigeria at my parents' church in Sanborn today. Not being great morning persons, we ventured to mom and dad's house last night for a sleep-over. Just walking in the house reminded me that as much as we have prepared, there are new corners and valleys we'll have to walk through as life continues without mom. Grief is a process and we've only begun. Megan

Monday, March 30, 2009 12:45 p.m.

Mindy and Sou had spent all of Saturday and most of Sunday with mom. Needing to take care of a few things at home, they ventured to Hull and planned to come back within a few hours. As Mike, dad and, Josh ran to get some molding material to make a print of mom's hand tonight, I was tempted to reach for the meaningless, trashy magazine that sat on the table. My mind was tired. As sacred as these last few weeks have been, I felt like running from sacred for a little while.

God's good senses urged me to press on and approach another sacred moment shared with my mom. Reaching for a book Rod Gorter, campus pastor at Dordt College, had dropped off a few weeks ago, I paged through and came upon the section "Confidence." Mindy had read through the entire book earlier in the day. Confidence seemed like something both mom and I needed to be reminded of this evening. "This looks like a good one mom," I said. And I began.

Hope springs eternal
in the heart of the child of God.
Nothing is ever hopeless
when your ways are committed to your Heavenly Father.
God's power is unlimited;
His goodness knows no measure;
His mercy knows no end.
No matter what news the day may bring,
you can accept it
with quiet confidence.
Nothing will ever happen to you
that is beyond
your Father's loving control.
Your Father
constantly watches over you.
Not one hair of your head
will fall to the ground
without His will!
Your confidence for the future
is built on an immovable foundation.

The Bible says . . .

"Those who trust in the Lord are like Mount Zion, which cannot be shaken but endures forever. As the mountains surround Jerusalem, so the LORD surrounds his people both now and forevermore" (Psalm 125:1-2). Jesus says, "Are not two sparrows sold for a penny? Yet not one of them will fall to the ground apart from the will of your Father. And even the very hairs of your head are all numbered. So don't be afraid; you are worth more than many sparrows" (Matthew 10:29-31).

After reading these words, I held mom's hand and prayed. I told God and mom how much I loved her and boldly asked God to show her something absolutely beautiful when she got to see Him for the first time. Seconds later, as I wondered and told mom how much I wish I could see what she'll see, mom quietly slipped away. And danced her way up to heaven. It was a peaceful moment and, for me, a reassuring departure from this earth and entrance into heaven.

The next few hours were meaningful as a family. We prayed and sang together, wondered together, and remembered an amazing wife and mother. And later, in honor of mom, I chugged a Diet Coke with grenadine. She had been waiting to do that for some time! Megan

Tuesday, March 31, 2009 10:07 a.m.

Visitation: Wednesday, April 1, 2009.
Funeral: Thursday, April 2, 2009. (On Cella's mother's birthday)

Thursday, April 2, 2009 12:20 p.m.

It's been a long few days, planning, preparing, and checking off all the things that needed to be done. Amazing, the effort it takes to pull together a funeral, especially following an intense three weeks taking care of a loved one.

Thanks for the love shown today and this evening. Between the gifts and visitors at visitation (estimated between 600-700 people) there was no doubt in our minds how special she was to many whose lives she touched. Megan

Monday, April 6, 2009 11:38 p.m.

It's hard to believe it's been a week since mom died. The first part of last week was filled to the brim with planning and preparing. I'm still surprised how little time a family has to let grief settle in with all the to-do lists a funeral entails. The latter part of the week gave us the opportunity to grieve, remember, and celebrate mom through visitation, the burial and memorial service in Sanborn, and the memorial service at Dordt College. We felt that all the events spoke very much about who mom was as a person, what she believed in, and how others felt about her. We left all the engagements filled with renewed hope that God was carrying us through and that God had carried mom through.

This last weekend we all started to catch up on rest, continued to answer questions our kids are asking, and started the transition to living without mom. For all of us, this transition is different. Having lived so far away, Mike and I didn't get to see mom on a daily basis. Mindy and her family did get to experience mom on a daily basis, whether that meant seeing each other in person or calling each other five times a day. Dad and Josh lived with mom day in and day out. Our tears will probably come at different times for each of us. We'll have different moments and reminders that urge within us a longing to have her here again. With that said, already we all feel deeply the lack of her presence. Loving deeply is amazing, but it brings deep pain as well.

My former manager at De Vos Children's Hospital has been encouraging me throughout this journey. She's walked alongside cancer and
end-of-life journeys with many pediatric patients and their families. She
often reminded me to keep looking out for the miracles, big and small,
that God would provide along the way. Sometimes we only attribute
cures and perfect-health-endings as miraculous workings from God. Jodi
helped keep me aware of the daily miracles and we definitely saw many of
these the past few weeks. None of the miracles defined being cured in the
way we all wanted mom to be healed, but they were miracles nonetheless.

I can vouch that we were probably the only family that considered
yesterday's winter wonderland a miracle. Even amidst the miracle we experienced, I found myself muttering under my breath, much like my
mother would do, complaining about the wretched April snowstorm that
covered this neck of the woods. Snow in April. I almost forgot how long
winter can linger in the Midwest.

Grandpa Jerry had been talking up his kid-size snowmobile to my
kids since our plans to be in the states materialized last October. Many
Nigerians heard about snowmobiles as Nico talked about it daily. We
figured our arrival to Iowa in mid-February meant for a safe promise to
our kids that they would get to ride a snowmobile once we arrived. Upon
arrival to Iowa, the snow melted. The weeks flew by snow-free and our
time soon became consumed with hospitals and loving mom to the very
end of her life. The snow stayed away long enough to provide for several
beautiful spring-like days when grandpa got to give all the kids a ride in
mom's blue convertible VW while at the Dougherty House. And then
comes yesterday, just after the burial and celebration of mom, snow cov-

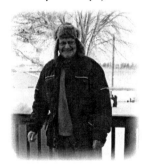

ered the earth and gave grandpa and the kids
a great day to play. I'm not sure who was more
excited yesterday, grandpa or the grandkids.
For my kids, it will be two and a half years
before they get to experience "winter" or snowmobiles again. (I hope anyway.) For grandpa,
this snow gave him a chance to play and laugh.
It provided for much fun and play. Riding in
the snowblower-tractor. Throwing snowballs.
Riding on the snowmobile. Kids often don't
let you forget that life continues. Yesterday was no exception. We were
thankful for the timing and blessing of the snow.

We may continue to post on mom's site for a little while. It doesn't feel right to shut it down yet. We have a few things we'll share concerning her funeral for people who live far away and weren't a part of her celebration of life. We know we'll for sure have a posting ready when Cella's newest grandbaby arrives . . . two weeks at the most.

I hope you are able to enjoy your big and small miracles today. Megan

Sunday, April 19, 2009 11:36 p.m.

Baby news? We've had lots of inquiries but no baby yet. That's right, we are still waiting. I've never been pregnant this long and it's provided for a very different experience! I'm not due until April 24; considering Amira was already five weeks old and Nico was two weeks old in my previous pregnancies, compared to their original due dates, we are surprised we are still waiting.

As much as we want to meet this little one, the extra time has been a bit of a blessing. The first week after the funeral was met with lots of sleep and catching up on things that had been neglected the weeks mom was in the hospital. This last week, we started the wonderful and difficult process of sorting through mom's things. Wanting to stay close to the Sioux Center Hospital until the baby arrives, Mindy, Mike, and I started in mom's office at Dordt College. We are finding all kinds of treasures! It's been at times wonderful as we find things that make us laugh or make us proud of her; other moments are difficult as we long to have her back instead of memories.

Grief is a process. A process where different phases are revisited often. We've all had good days and we've all had bad days. Amira's been compared with Aunt Mindy in her childhood days of dressing. Mom always got a kick out of hearing the latest concoction. When Amira came up the stairs for her first soccer game last week, decked out in her red shorts, green and yellow top, and white socks pulled all the way up through her shorts resembling two skinny leg casts, it hurt not to call mom to share Amira's ensemble and to hear mom's jovial laughter in response.

Dad says Sunday's are the most difficult for him. Sunday was their day. Mom was typically running around for something she was doing for church in the morning or evening service. The rest of the day was either filled with family gatherings or lounging at home. Dad loved seeing mom use her gifts. It's been a difficult process to go back to their home church as there are so many memories of mom buzzing around church, adding to worship. The entire day is very lonely without her. We are very proud of how proactive dad has been in his grieving process. As proactive as he has been, it doesn't take the pain out of walking through these days and weeks.

We appreciate your prayers for strength and wisdom and guidance as we continue to walk the path of grief.

We'll be in touch with baby news—I hope sooner than later! Megan

Thursday, April 23, 2009 12:59 p.m.

It's a GIRL!

Stella Egheosasere (pronounced eh OH suh say) quickly arrived last night! (More on her name later . . . .) We arrived at the hospital at 6:15 p.m. and met little Stella at 7:42 p.m. She took her time, but when she finally decided to come, she wasted no time. She weighed seven pounds four ounces and was 21 1/2 inches long.

Wednesday, April 29, 2009 2:21 a.m.

Mom always made us promise we would never name a baby Cella or Marcella. She was never fond of her name. The week before mom and dad left for Mexico, we dined at the local Jay's Restaurant in Sanborn. While we were waiting for our food, mom whispered, wondering what we would name this baby. The boy name was quickly approved but I knew I'd need to do some explaining and pleading with her on our girl name. Stella Egheosasere was quickly approved . . . far away enough from Cella for mom and close enough for me! Egheosasere comes from another spe-

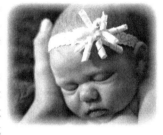

cial person in our life. Eghe (egg eh) lived with us in Nigeria for two years and Grand Rapids for two years. She quickly became part of our family. Mom made many surprise trips to Michigan to see her in plays and attend her graduation ceremonies. Not only is Eghe special to us, but the meaning of her full name could not be more fitting for this season in our life. Egheosasere means God's time is best. Mike and I were scheduled to come home a year from now. Because of Stella's little growing life, an early "home service" was approved and planned. Little did we know all the events that would unfold upon our coming home. We could have never orchestrated this time if we had tried. God's time is not always ours, but there's no doubt in my mind that it is best.

Stella had her first sleep-over at grandpa's this weekend. She wasn't the best of company as she welcomed herself by peeing in his bed. We're not sure how the diaper got missed but the bedsheet filled.

Most of us are still a bit surprised Stella is a girl. For some reason, most of us thought she would be a he. In some ways, it has made grieving a lot harder—saying her name so close to mom's. Sorting through the darling clothes mom bought for Amira . . . she LOVED to shop! Having flashbacks of Amira's first few months of life when we lived with mom and dad, again in transit from life in Nigeria, has made us miss mom much more. But it's also made it easier. It's forced me to remember mom in very real ways. And it has forced me to face her absence. Her presence is missed in indescribable ways and at the same time is felt more than ever. Whether we have good days of remembering mom in laughter and in other wonderful ways or in very rough days of not knowing what to do or where to turn, we are all taking one moment at a time.

The new life doesn't replace Cella's, but Stella's coming softens the loss.

> For everything there is a season . . .
> and a time for every matter under heaven:
> a time to be born, and a time to die;
> a time to plant, and a time to pluck up what is planted;
> a time to kill, and a time to heal;
> a time to break down, and a time to build up;
> a time to weep, and a time to laugh;
> a time to mourn, and a time to dance;
> a time to cast away stones, and a time to gather stones together;
> a time to embrace, and a time to refrain from embracing;
> a time to seek, and a time to lose;
> a time to keep, and a time to cast away;
> a time to tear, and a time to sew;
> a time to keep silence, and a time to speak;
> a time to love, and a time to hate;
> a time for war, and a time for peace. (Ecclesiastes 3:1-8 ESV)

. . . embracing each season as it comes, moment by moment.
Megan

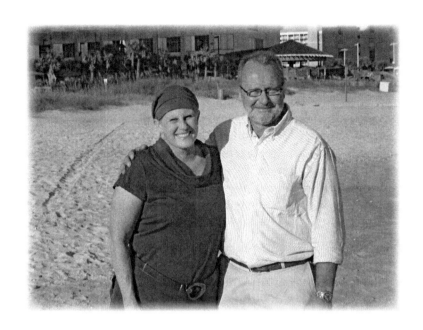

POSTSCRIPT

Marcella Faye (Cleveringa) Bosma was born in Canton, South Dakota, on September 26, 1953, to Roger and Esther (Vanden Bosch) Cleveringa. Cella's delight in learning started while growing up on a farm near Rock Valley, Iowa. Her mother strongly encouraged reading and taught her much at an early age. As a child, she was curious, wanting to know how to cook, sew, and drive the tractor and help with farm chores. She had a passion for singing and making music. For her elementary and secondary education, she attended Rock Valley Christian School, Inwood Christian School, and Hull Western Christian High School.

Cella's active lifestyle began when she was a young high school student. From sports to music to committees, these many activities no doubt prepared her for the busy lifestyle on which she thrived all her life.

Cella married her high school sweetheart and life-long storyteller, Jerry Lee Bosma, on December 30, 1973, at First Christian Reformed Church in Rock Valley, Iowa. As a couple, they lived in Utah for two years then resided in Sanborn, Iowa, for the rest of their married life where they welcomed three children and eventually six grandchildren into their lives. Family was always a priority. Cella's love for children and grandchildren was evident in her own family activities and reached deep into the community. She was an active member of Sanborn CRC, playing organ for worship services and teaching Sunday school, determined to be faithful at nurturing students of all ages in the Christian community. Together, Jerry and Cella taught Sunday School and Young Adult Bible Studies. For eleven years Cella's combined love for children, service, and cultures led to her passionate involvement in service-learning groups to Cary, Mississippi, assisted the last six years by Jerry.

Cella received her bachelor of arts degree from Dordt College in 1984, masters of education from Northwestern College in 1992, and was pursuing the Ed.D. degree at the University of South Dakota. Her delight for learning flowed into practical, biblical teaching. As a classroom teacher, she taught second grade at Sanborn Christian for eleven years and fifth grade at Sheldon Christian for seven years. Cella was an education professor at Dordt College since 2000, teaching seven different courses ranging from Introduction to Education to Teaching Social Studies in the Elementary Classroom to Philosophy of Education; in addition to supervising and mentoring countless student teachers. In 2007 she received the alumni-selected John Calvin Award for excellence in teaching. She also was a leader in Northwest Iowa Reading Council, the

Association for Supervision and Curriculum Development, and Heartland Christian Teacher's Convention.

Cella loved life. She lived it full and fast, from her teaching style to the very way she walked and talked. Her enthusiasm for living could be seen as she worked her flower garden, read to her grandchildren, made music, promoted education, and traveled the world. One of her students once, with some hyperbole, characterized one of her classes thus: "She came into class talking and did not take a breath until the class ended fifty minutes later." She was also known as the teacher who always had time to guide and encourage students who came to her for help. She had an exuberant style of teaching and never tired until medication for her cancer occasionally sapped her energy in her last two years of teaching. Her enthusiasm spilled into the lives of her family, friends, peers, colleagues, and students.

Cella will be sorely missed by Jerry, her husband of thirty-five years; her son Josh; two daughters and their husbands and children: Megan and Mike Ribbens, and children, Amira, Nico, and Stella; Mindy and Souvanna Baccam, and children Kobi, Bailey, and Miles Baccam; parents Roger and Esther Cleveringa; siblings Norm and LaDonna Cleveringa, Marcia and Lee Rozeboom; and many other relatives and friends.

-Dr. Mike Vanden Bosch and family of Cella

SELECTED GUEST BOOK ENTRIES—
MARCH/APRIL 2009

"Remembering you guys in prayer today as you celebrate Cella's life. We have all been blessed to have her touch our lives in someway that will live on in all of us forever." Brian g.

"Cella was such a vibrant, vivacious spirit that things livened up when she was near." Glenn d.j.

"Cella is the most special person and I am so very thankful to have known her and that two of my children were blessed to have had her for a teacher at Sheldon Christian." Sue z.

"I got to know Cella when she came down to Rehoboth to supervise student teachers. She and I were immediate soul mates. Her humor and energy filled the room. Her encouragement and passion spurred her students to improvement and success. Cella didn't live on the surface. She touched souls." Short h.

"I still remember walking into Ed. 101 and being welcomed by Cella's constant smile. She has been a huge inspiration to me. Her love for others is evident. She went out of her way to show me and many others that we mattered to her. She is a role model for me as I think about becoming a teacher." Michaela g.

". . . This morning the Dordt College community gathered in chapel and spent an extended time in prayer for you and others affected by this death. There was an atmosphere of grief in letting go of a dearly beloved colleague, teacher, and sister in Christ. . . . We rejoiced in the life and faith of Cella who has touched many of us in a lasting way. We will miss her deeply." Rod g.

"I had Mrs. Bosma as a second/third grade teacher. My favorite memory? She used to pull out our teeth—literally. When we had the slightest wiggle to one of our primary teeth, we would run to Mrs. Bosma and beg her to pull it out—and she would. She is truly an amazing lady." Katie j.

"I had the privilege to have Cella for two education classes at Dordt. I loved both classes and wish I could've had her for more classes. She was so enthusiastic for what she was teaching and it showed. No matter how Cella was feeling, she had energy and a big smile." Megan v.e.

"I have many special memories of [Cella] and I am thankful for many aspects of her. . . . You summed it up beautifully, Megan, that your mom has made many people feel that she is like their own mother, sister, daughter, best friend . . . just by being herself and having such a presence about her." Michelle v.

"Cella is a great woman and will be dearly missed by all. No matter what was going on, she always had a kind word and a smile on her face. She always made me feel better when I was feeling down or homesick. She has that kind of effect on everyone." Jessica s.

"May you find strength in each other and in God to know that He is taking into his kingdom a wonderful new angel. . . . In the six years I have had the privilege of knowing Cella, she has done more in her short life than most can even aspire to do. She has inspired me and just reflecting on her life keeps me going." Nicole c.

"I first met Cella as my prof in Gen. 100 at Dordt. As my semester unraveled, I began to doubt whether I had made a good decision to come to Dordt. . . . found comfort, though, in one person—Cella—my prof, advisor, and friend. I looked forward to each class I had with her in Gen. 100. God's love was overflowing through Cella. . . . She was encouraging, kind, gentle, patient, and my comic relief . . . in class and in meetings. . . . She captures Philippians 2:1-11. Kyle r.

"You don't know me—I was given this site by a friend. . . . I am overwhelmed by how Christ-honoring this site is. . . . You and the people who are posting on this guest book are always pointing to Christ and . . . the real hope we have in our God." Paul h.

"You are being uplifted in our hearts and minds, even from as far away as China! I was one of Cella's students at Dordt—impacted by the passion with which Cella taught, and how she instilled that love of the Father in us, her students." Jolene d.

"I will always remember Prof. Bosma as a strong woman who walked down the hallway with confidence in her step and a bright smile on her face. She was a great blessing to the Dordt community." Sarah g.

"Oh, how we all ache and miss her already. She was a true gem . . . the precious and rare kind that is priceless. How proud you must be of her, of the legacy she has left behind." Kevin v.m.

LaVergne, TN USA
04 February 2010
172088LV00004B/1/P